THE ROAD TO A LEANER YOU

Permanently Lose 10, 20, 50, 100+ Pounds the Healthy Way

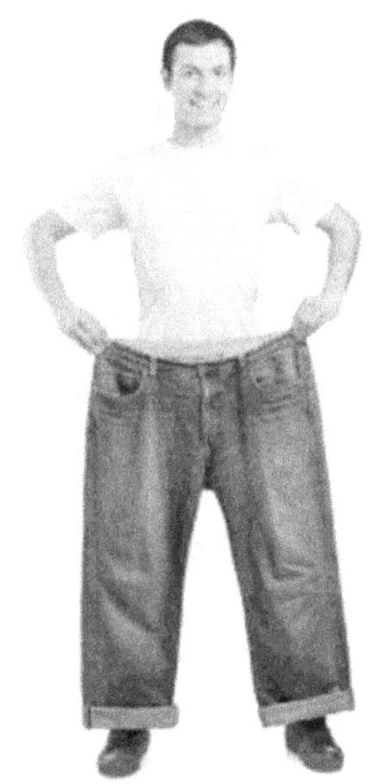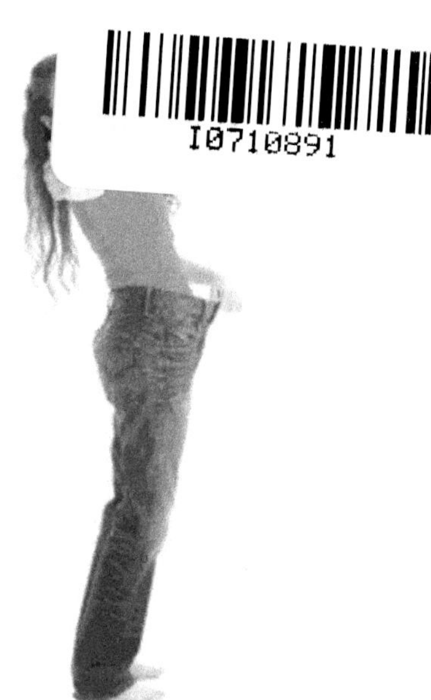

Cary Cavitt

Author & Speaker

To book a speaking engagement please visit us at
www.roadtobetterhealth.net

ISBN-13:
978-1983599811

ISBN-10:
1983599816

Looking for a fun and educational health seminar for your next event?

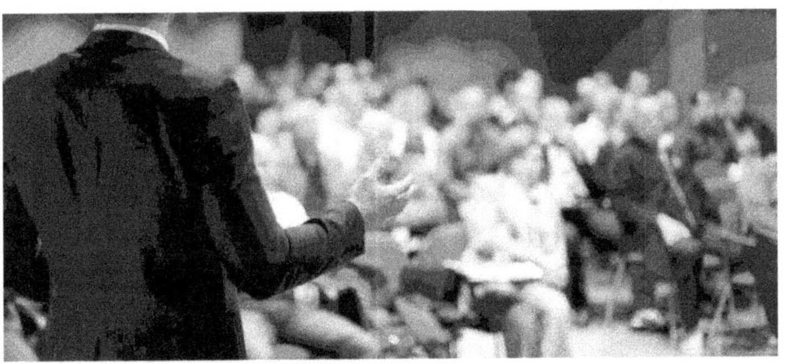

If you would like to book Cary at your next meeting on the topic of becoming healthier, then please visit us at:

www.roadtobetterhealth.net

Whether your next event revolves around offering a health seminar for your workplace, upcoming expo or conference, church or civic club, or any other type of social group, our *Road to Better Health Seminars* are a perfect fit to educate your audience on how to feel better, lose weight, and think clearer. Contact us today at www.roadtobetterhealth.net.

This book is dedicated to those who are tired of carrying around extra weight.

Take courage and stay the course. Get sugar and processed foods completely out of your life and permanent weight loss will occur.

My advice is to learn to eat REAL FOOD. Real food does not have ingredients. Real food is ingredients.

Remember, eating does not make you fat. Eating bad food does.

- Cary Cavitt

Other authored health book

www.roadtobetterhealth.net

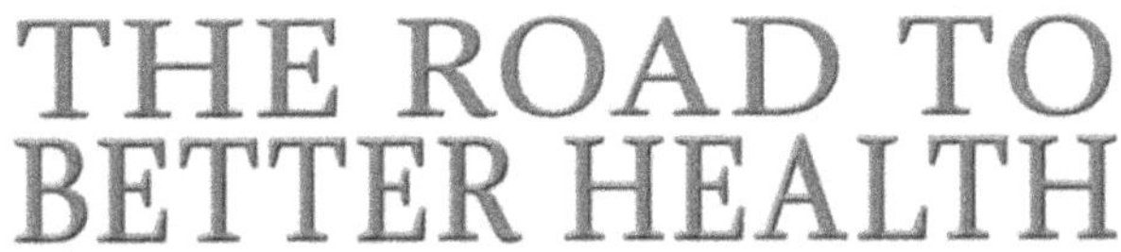

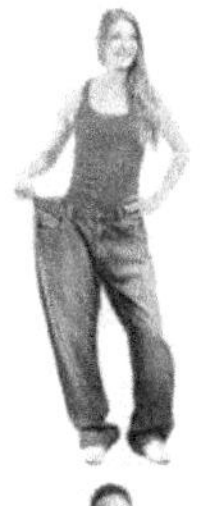
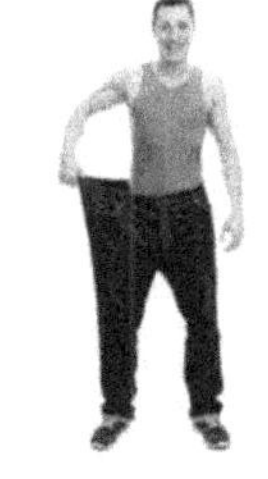
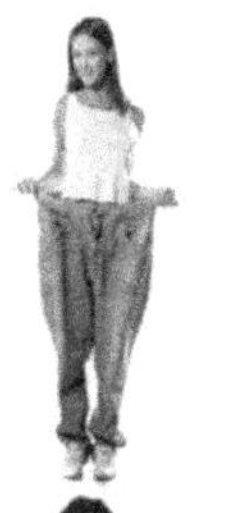
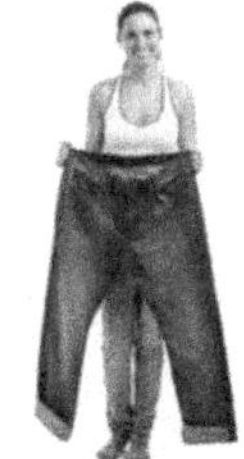
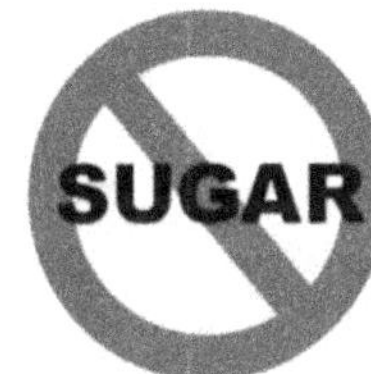

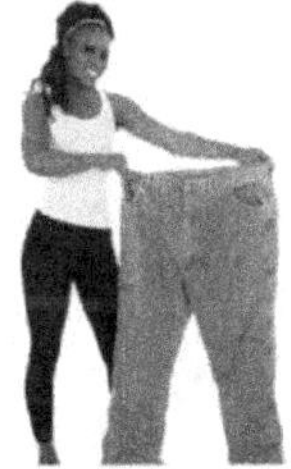
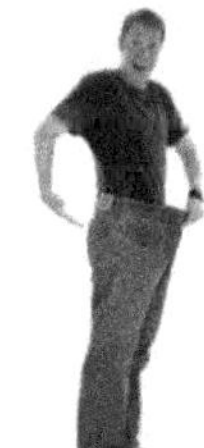
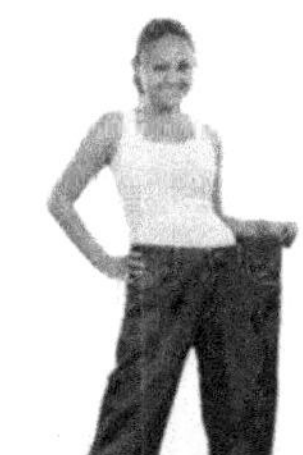
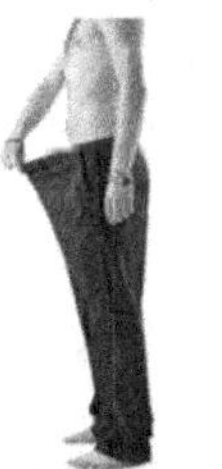

Table of Contexts

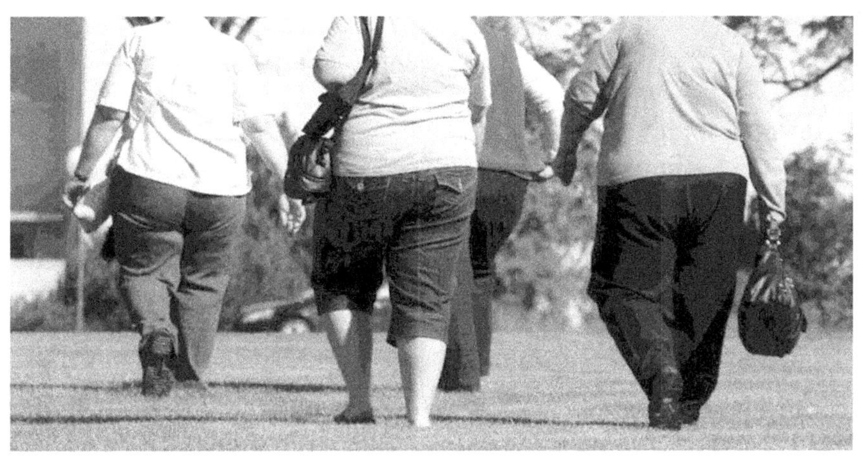

Introduction

Trim & Fit... It is abnormal today in our overweight society

We live in a day and age where being overweight is normal and being trim & fit is abnormal. Strange but true.

There was a time when the majority of people within our society were actually trim and fit. Grab any pre-1970 picture of a group of people and you will be hard pressed to see two overweight people in the same picture within any of these old photos.

I believe that we would all agree that there is a serious weight problem in America as statistics are telling us that 2 out of 3 adults are either overweight or obese. This truly is a health issue that needs to be addressed.

And with so much information out there the question is *why do the majority of people fail when it comes to losing weight?*

As a follow up to my first health book entitled *The Road to Better Health*, I will again offer 53 easy to understand tips for becoming healthier and losing weight permanently.

I personally believe losing weight has everything to do with learning to eat REAL FOOD that will keep your insulin low.

Plain and simple fact: We have become a fat nation due in large part to the abundance of cheap producing processed foods that make up the majority of grocery store products (sorry TV dinners, pastas, and bread products).

In our present society go out anywhere and you are sure to see that the majority of people walking around you are either overweight or obese. And on the other end of the spectrum, it is a rare occurrence to see a person over 40 (or is it 30?) who is trim and fit.

I personally do not put all of the blame on the shoulders of overweight people. *What I do put the majority of the blame on is the overwhelming amount of garbage food that is readily available at your friendly grocery store.*

My heart goes out to those who are fighting a weight issue simply because carrying all of that extra weight is unhealthy and opens the door to so many diseases. Life truly is much more difficult for overweight people and a simple task like walking in the park can become overwhelming.

My one advice that I would offer to anyone who is fighting an overweight issue is to stop eating sugar and processed foods. This in turn will keep your bodies' insulin level low throughout the day, thus allowing body fat to be burned as energy.

Give your body REAL FOOD and trust me when I say that your weight will begin to drop in a healthy and timely manner.

More than likely your overweight problem has everything to do with years of *poor food choices.* So are you ready to let that leaner person inside of you come out? I sincerely hope so. Maybe it is finally time to make a 180° turnabout. Remember…

Extreme times *require* **extreme measures.**

May the following 53 quick tips assist you in your journey.

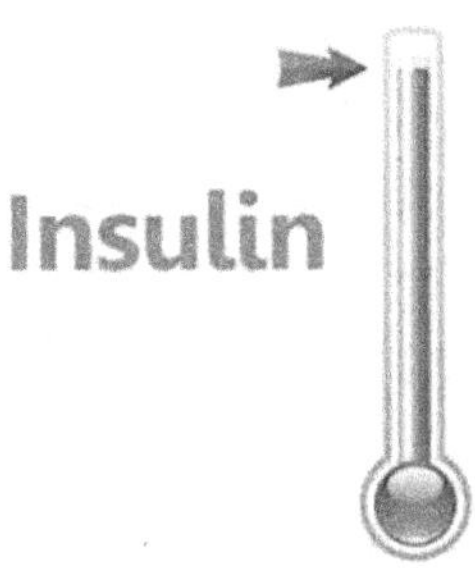

What happens when our **insulin** levels are **high?**

Tip #1
Keep your insulin low... The most important tip

If I were cornered and asked directly what I would consider to be the #1 HEALTHY and PERMANENT way to lose weight, this would be my response without hesitation:

"Eat foods that keep your insulin low, period."

In my personal opinion, understanding this key point will be a GAME CHANGER for anyone wanting to become both healthier and leaner.

My belief is that the reason that you may have never heard about the importance of insulin is because most doctors and nutritionists are still stuck in the science of the 1960's and honestly have no clear understanding on this subject.

Another reason that you may have never heard about keeping your insulin low is that there is NO MONEY TO BE MADE in this *(sorry Jenny Craig, Nutrisystem, and Marie Osmond)*.

Without losing you by getting technical, here is the only thing that you need to understand:

When you eat foods (think REAL FOODS like meats and veggies) that keep your insulin low, you are now allowing your body to burn fat as your daily energy source.

In other words, the fat on your body is now allowed to be used as energy. This of course is the key for losing that fat on your belly and waistline.

But when you eat foods that raise your insulin *(sorry pastas, potatoes, bread, and sugar lovers)*, you will never be able to tap into your fat as an energy source.

Instead you will be spending your days using carbs and sugar as your main energy source. This is why the majority of people cannot and will never lose weight. The key in weight loss is to tap into your body fat as the main energy source.

Also, living with a high insulin state becomes the direct cause of so many chronic diseases. This is why keeping your insulin low throughout the day is the key to optimal health as well as losing fat from your body.

In closing, there is a 26-minute video on YouTube that completely opened my eyes to the dangers of high insulin levels and what it does to a person's body.

Simply type into YouTube *The Root of Modern Illness - High Insulin* as it explains the damaging effects of having high insulin in your body.

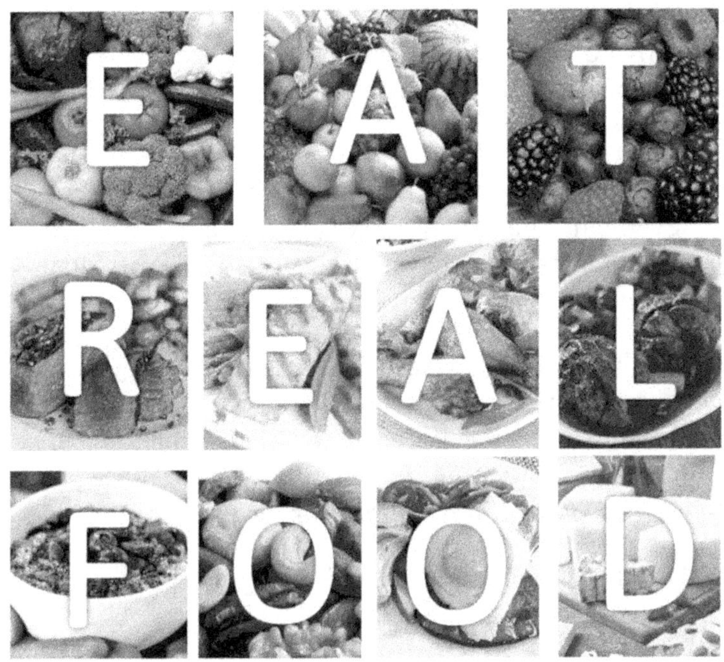

Tip #2
Eat REAL FOOD... The 2nd most important tip

Learning to eat REAL FOOD is the 2nd most important tip that I would offer to anyone who is tired of living a life in an overweight body.

Keeping your insulin low throughout the day is the most important tip, and eating REAL FOOD will allow this to occur. Let me give you a clear understanding of what REAL FOOD actually is.

If I were to give an educational tour in a typical grocery store, I would first of all point out that approximate 80% of everything in the store is what I would classify as processed food, or what I call FAKE FOOD *(that most of us have been eating all of our lives)*.

This fake food is usually manufactured in a windowless factory and typically comes in a box, bag, can, or is frozen. You will also notice that the majority of shoppers in the store have filled their carts with these types of foods.

These fake foods have very little nutritional value. What they do offer is eventual weight gain and weird internal diseases simply because our bodies were never designed to live off of this stuff *(sorry Doritos)*.

Also, these processed foods are made to taste really yummy by the laboratory scientists who love to add sugar and strange ingredients that are hard to pronounce. *We need to remember that this is all about big profits for the food companies, and what it does to the customer's overall health is of little concern to them.*

I have always said that if Abe Lincoln did not eat it, then more than likely it is a processed fake food.

On the other hand, most of the food that 'ol Abe would have ate is more than likely REAL FOOD. So a good question to ask prior to eating anything is whether or not our friendly 16th President would have eaten it.

Listen carefully. Our body craves REAL FOOD *(hello steak and broccoli),* and rebels when we give it processed food by eventually making us fat and sick.

If we genuinely want to become healthier, then we need to stop eating the majority of foods in our friendly grocery store that come in a box, bag, can, or is frozen.

And again, simply ask yourself if 'ol Abe would have eaten it.

Sorry corn dogs.

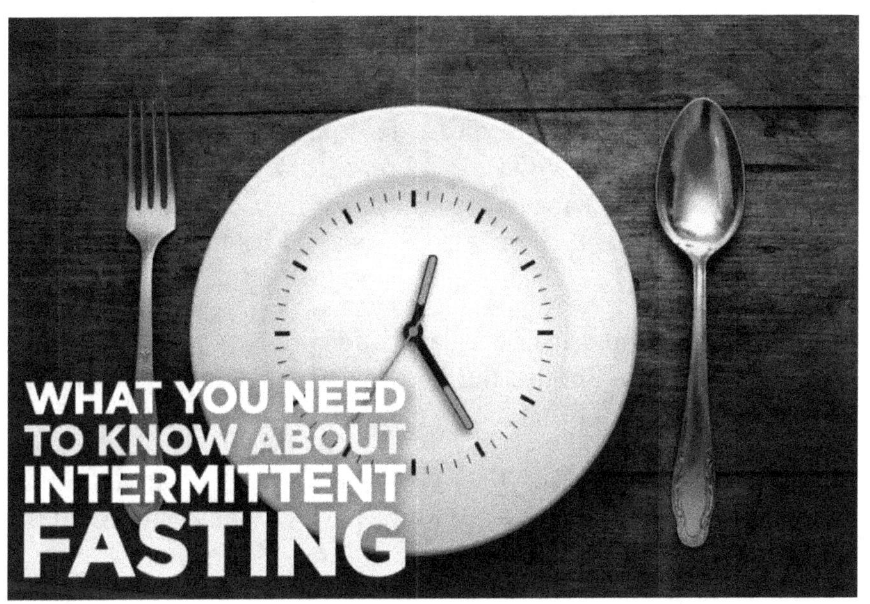

Tip #3
Intermittent Fasting... The 3rd most important tip

Here is what I would list as the three most important keys to losing weight permanently:

#1 Simply keep your insulin low throughout the day
#2 Learn to eat REAL FOOD and divorce FAKE FOOD
#3 Make intermittent fasting a daily part of your life

Let's focus on intermittent fasting.

I cannot think of anything healthier for your body than getting into the habit of intermittent fasting. If you are serious about wanting to feel better and become leaner, then you need to do this.

Not only are you allowing your body to get rest from constantly stuffing down food, but intermittent fasting is a great way to permanently lose weight by burning fat on your body as the main source for energy.

As humans we were never meant to consistently be stuffing our bellies with food. *It really is abnormal to always be eating.* We live in a culture where cheap unhealthy food is everywhere. In reality the only time that we seriously should be eating is when we are actually hungry.

But due to our three meals a day belief *(or is it now five?),* our culture has the mindset that our body needs to constantly be stuffed with food or else we could die of starvation.

So many people go all their lives without ever giving their digestive system a rest, and we wonder why the majority of adults are living off of prescription pills.

I personally believe that a high percentage of people never truly experience real hunger simply because we have so much cheap food available. It seems that most people are constantly feeding their faces with processed, cheap food. No wonder we have an overweight society.

So let's get back to why intermittent fasting is so good for your health. Let's first define exactly what it is:

"Intermittent fasting is not eating anywhere between 16 to 20 hours each day."

In other words, you are giving your digestive system some much needed rest each day *as well as allowing your body to burn fat on your hips and belly as the primary energy source during the fasting state (a really good thing).*

Some of you may be thinking that not eating for 16-20 hours per day is unhealthy or could cause starvation. Nothing could be further from the truth.

The absolute easiest way to intermittent fast is to *simply STOP EATING BREAKFAST each morning.* Even though you may have been eating breakfast since you were one years old, trust me when

I say that it really is not necessary.

Tony the Tiger and Captain Crunch have basically brainwashed our society into believing that eating a breakfast is the most important meal of the day.

In my opinion it is all a fabricated lie brought to you by the zillion dollars a year food industry that wants you to stuff your face every morning with their processed junk food.

Simply skip breakfast every morning and you will be intermittent fasting!

Here are 3 choices for your eating window:

BEGINNER: 16 Hour Intermittent Fast...
Eat only between 12:00 pm and 8:00 pm.

ADVANCED: 18 Hour Intermittent Fast...
Eat only between 12:00 pm and 6:00 pm.

SUPER ADVANCED: 20 Hour Intermittent Fast...
Eat only between 2:00 pm and 6:00 pm.

The first week or so will be difficult as your belly will continue to protest. *But be assured that the protest will not be due to starvation.* The belly protest will be more about wanting food in the morning since it has been a habit that you have had for decades.

And remember that as you begin to eat REAL FOOD during your eating window, you will be more satisfied and full for a much longer duration of time.

One of the major reasons that most people wake up hungry is because their daily diets consist primarily of carb loaded processed foods (which only satisfies hunger for a short period).

By eating REAL FOOD (think meat and healthy fats), you will begin to wake up less hungry, and waiting until noon or later to eat will soon become a breeze.

If you are serious about losing weight, then I would highly recommend intermittent fasting as one of the top three keys to losing fat.

By making it a habit to fast 16+ hours a day, not only will you allow your body to rest from the constant need to digest food, but this longer resting period will allow the stored fat on your hips and belly to be burned for energy. *This is the real secret to healthy and permanent weight loss.*

Try intermittent fasting and within one week your brain will not only be able to focus so much better, but your whole body will begin to lose unwanted fat and feel so much lighter.

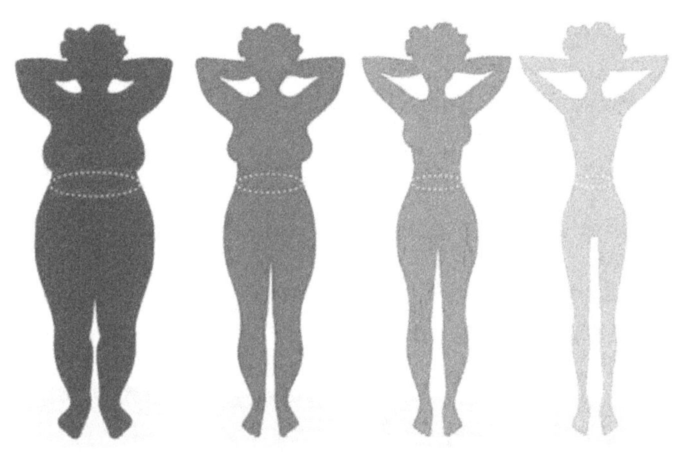

Tip #4
5 simple questions to lose weight and become healthy

Get all 5 questions right and it will show that you have left the flawed advice of the lab scientists with white lab coats from the 1960's.

#1 How can you permanently get rid of that belly you hate looking at in a mirror and try to hide it with clothing?

A. Go to the gym daily and do 8,350 crunches for 9 months.

B. Borrow your great grandmother's girdle and wear it all day.

C. Learn to keep your insulin low with REAL FOODS.

D. Buy those diet pills you saw at Walgreens on the clearance rack.

If you picked C. you are 100% correct. Trust me when I say that you will get leaner by just eating real food.

#2 Why would I recommend skipping breakfast and do

intermittent fasting?

    A. To save money since Captain Crunch is getting expensive.

    B. So that you don't have to do the dishes in the morning.

    C. So you will have time to sleep in longer.

    D. To allow your body a longer time to burn fat as your source of energy.

If you picked D. you are 100% correct.

#3 What group of cooking oils would I only use?

    A. Butter, Olive Oil, Coconut Oil, Lard

    B. Crisco, Margarine, Vegetable Oil, Canola Oil, and any other manufactured oil in a clear bottle.

If you picked A. you are 100% correct. *(I would HIGHLY RECOMMEND throwing away anything on list B immediately).*

#4 The average person in America consumes approximately 150 pounds of this "toxic poison to the body" annually. What is it?

A. Sodium
B. Sugar
C. Fake Commercial Oils
D. Monster Drinks

If you picked B. you are 100% correct.

#5 If I wanted to lose 10, 20, 50, or 100+ pounds I would personally do what?

    A. Join the Jenny Craig, Weight Watchers, or Nutrisystem program for life even though it will be expensive in the long run.

    B. Eat between 800 -1200 calories a day, feel miserable, weak, and fragile all day. Sure it is super unhealthy and impossible to sustain, but isn't that the only way?

C. Learn to keep my insulin low, live an intermittent fasting lifestyle, eat REAL FOOD, eat until I am full and satisfied *(like we humans were meant to do),* and avoid the majority of boxed, bagged, canned, and frozen foods that are made in a basement factory somewhere in New York City.

D. Try the latest silly diet such as the *Hollywood Grapefruit Miracle Diet,* the *Marshmallow Slim Diet,* or the *Snickers Candy Bar Wonder Diet.* Or better yet, go get my stomach stapled as that sounds like a healthy move.

If you picked C. you are 100% correct. Since I eat real food I am never hungry in the morning and can easily skip breakfast. But since the majority of overweight people live off of processed foods, they always tend to wake up in the morning starving for a fat producing bagel or blueberry muffin.

In summary, the majority of overweight people will continue to stay fat because of these reasons:

- They eat foods that always spike their insulin.

- They are brainwashed into thinking they will die or become unhealthy by skipping breakfast.

- They consume trans fats and fake oils (which are terrible).

- They are addicted to sugar and don't even know it (sad but true).

- They continue to follow silly diets that are nothing more than scams.

"Learn to keep my insulin low, live an intermittent fasting lifestyle, eat REAL FOOD, eat until I am full and satisfied (like we humans were meant to do), and avoid the majority of boxed, bagged, canned, and frozen foods that are made in a basement factory somewhere in New York City."

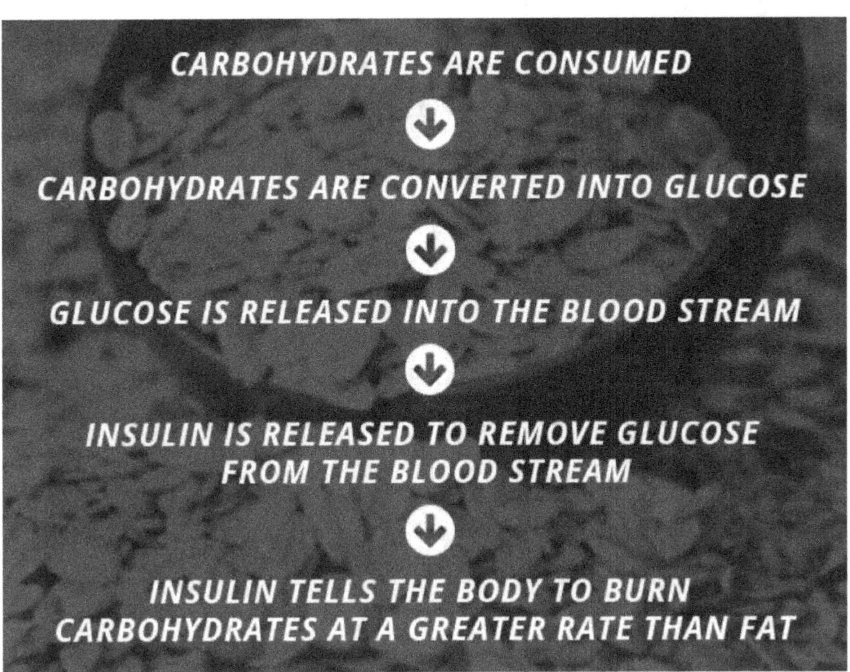

Tip #5
Why you have never heard about keeping insulin low

If keeping your insulin low is one of the major keys in losing unwanted weight, then why have I never heard about it?

Great question and here is the simple answer:

"Because there is no money to be made in it."

The weight loss industry is a multi-billion dollar operation and a whole lot of money is made by all of these calorie-restricted TV diet programs out there.

Trust me when I say that Ms. Jenny Craig or Ms. Weight Watchers *will never tell you about keeping your insulin low* as the permanent solution to getting rid of your belly and hips. Instead they will ship you *expensive low calorie unhealthy food in a box* that will instantly spike your insulin (which is not a good thing).

If all of these very profitable TV diet programs started teaching people about keeping insulin low, they would soon be out of business and not be able to scam, I mean sell naïve customers their unhealthy low calorie processed food.

Begin to live an intermittent fasting lifestyle *(just Google to learn more),* and learn to keep your insulin low with real food, and you will soon be heading out to your favorite clothing store to get a smaller wardrobe.

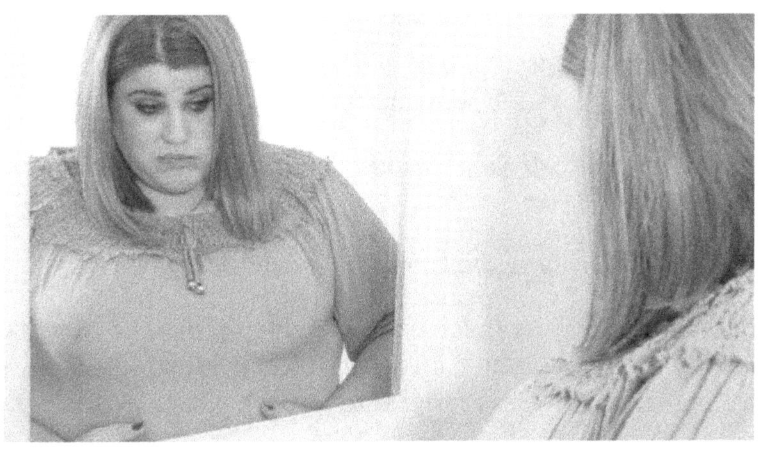

Tip #6
Why most overweight people will never lose weight

One of the main reasons why most overweight people will remain the same for years *(or decades)* is simply because they cannot believe that there is a leaner person inside waiting to escape.

For years you have looked into a mirror and have just accepted that this is the way that you will look for the rest of your life. This is completely wrong thinking, and more than likely keeping you from becoming a healthier, leaner person.

It may also be hard to imagine that you can actually lose all of that weight and get back to how much you may have weighed years earlier.

But I am here to tell you that you can do a total makeover and lose that weight permanently.

Please do not believe the person in the mirror looking back at you and silently whispering in your ear that this is how you are going to look or feel for the rest of your life.

There is a leaner and healthier person inside of you if you can only start to believe that *weight can and will come off* by understanding these two major keys for permanent weight loss:

> *#1 Learn to keep your insulin low throughout the day (with real foods).*

> *#2 Make intermittent fasting a daily part of your life.*

It does not matter how much extra weight you may be carrying on your body today. Simply learn about the above two tips and watch as that person in the mirror begins to lose weight.

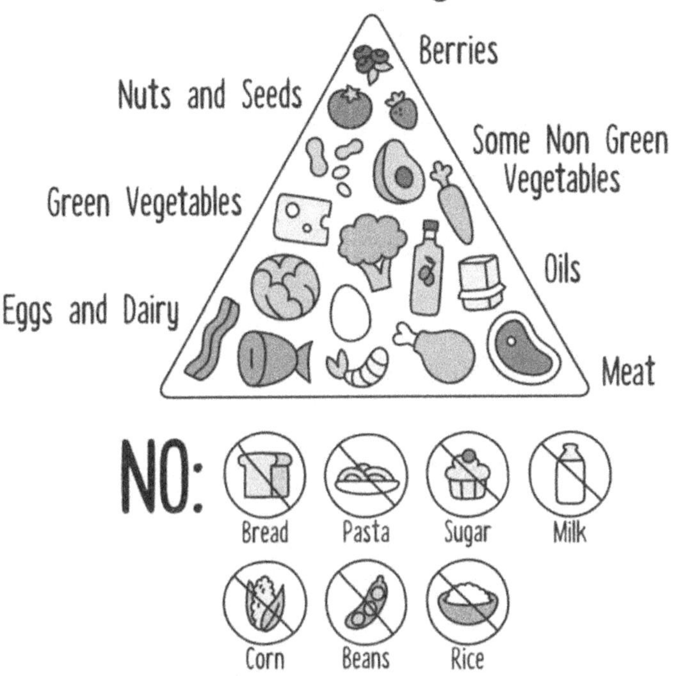

Tip #7
Foods that will make you both fat and lean

Below are two lists. The first list is part of the Standard American Diet (SAD Diet) that the majority of your neighborhood follows, and hence is overweight. These processed foods really never satisfy and that is the reason that you may constantly be hungry and stay overweight.

The second list is foods that not only will keep you full for a really long time, but are what I call REAL FOOD *(not made in a basement factory somewhere in New York City)*. Eat these foods and you will begin seeing a leaner person in the mirror.

SOME FOODS THAT WILL CONTINUE TO MAKE YOU FAT:

- All Pastas (sorry pasta lovers and mac & cheese fans)

- Potatoes (your body sees it as a lump of sugar)

- Boxed Cereals (spikes insulin which is bad)

- Fruit Juices (even 100% juice which is terrible for you)

- All Store & Restaurant Breads (Panera bread makes you fat)

- ALL Muffins, Bagels and All Baked Goods (sorry nutty donut lovers)

- Corn (including popcorn / we feed cows corn to fatten them up)

- Soda Pop & Majority of Other Sugar Laced Beverages (should be illegal)

- Rice and Beans (spikes insulin which is why you are overweight)

- Desserts, Ice Cream, Candy, ALL Chips in a bag (instant fat)

- Majority of Fast Food Restaurants (95% of menu terrible for hips)

- Pizza (sorry fans, but the bread they use will expand your belly)

- Fake Cooking Oils (Crisco and its fellow cohorts)

- Any Other Food That Spikes the Insulin

SOME FOODS THAT WILL MAKE YOU LEAN (keeps insulin low)

- Steak and Hamburger *(eat the fat as it will not make you fat or give you a heart attack, since sugar is the real culprit)*

- Most Other Meats

- Eggs and Bacon

- 100% Butter / Real Cheese

- Veggies and Salads *(love broccoli)*

- Coconut Oil and Olive Oil

- Peanut Butter *(a spoonful won't harm you & a great treat!)*

- Any Other Food That Keeps the Insulin Low

Remember that approximately 80% of the foods *(think boxed, bagged, canned, or frozen)* at your friendly grocery store will expand your belly and hips. I primarily stay in the veggie and meat section of grocery stores where there is REAL FOOD.

"Remember that approximately 80% of the foods (think boxed, bagged, canned, or frozen) at your friendly grocery store will expand your belly and hips."

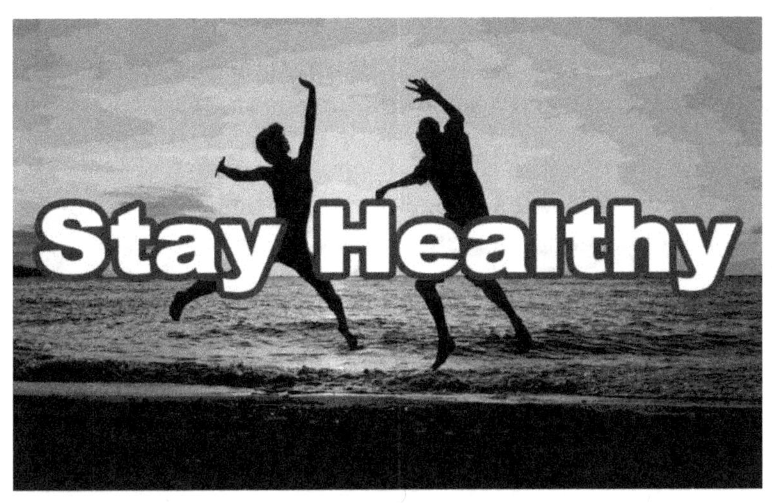

Tip #8
10 keys to stay lean and healthy

If someone were to ask me what they needed to do to stay lean and healthy, I would give them the following 10 answers:

#1 Keep your insulin low by eating REAL FOOD *(sorry corn dogs and pasta)*

#2 Intermittent fast everyday (just eat between 12-8 pm)

#3 Get enough sleep every night (I try to get 8+ hours)

#4 Avoid 80% of grocery store products *(think box, bag, can, frozen)*

#5 Do a simple exercise program 3-4 times a week

#6 Get a stand-up desk to work at

#7 Avoid 99.9% of canned or bottled beverages

#8 Just DIVORCE all forms of sugars *(it is toxin to your body)*

#9 Get stress out of your life (produces a big belly)

#10 Inform yourself with the information and videos on my educational website **www.roadtobetterhealth.net**.

Follow the above 10 tips and not only will you feel better within one week, but you will soon get back that high school weight that you thought was gone forever.

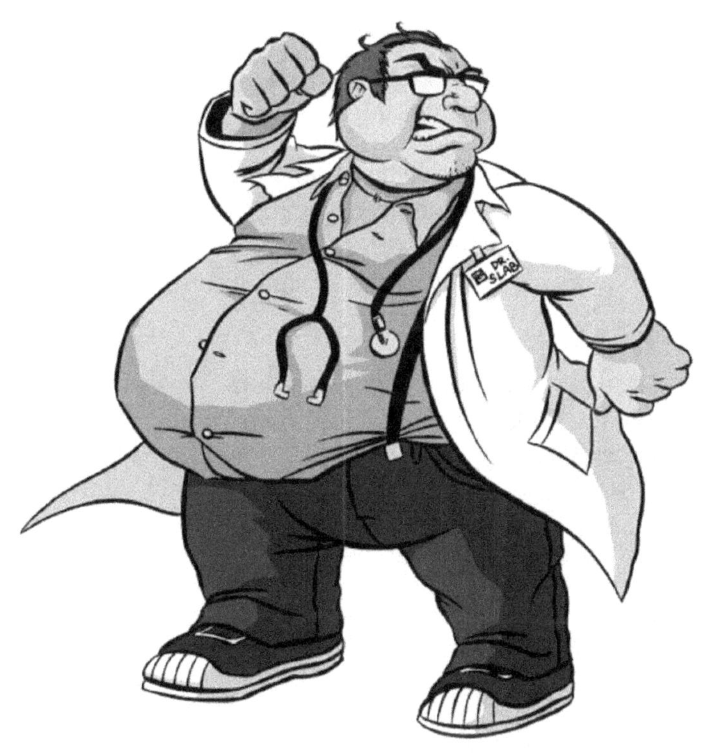

Tip #9
Why are you still listening to your overweight doctor?

Not to be rude, but if your doctor is out of shape or overweight, and offers you counsel on being healthier or losing weight, I personally would run from his or her advice on this specific topic.

Sure they may be a specialist in their field of endeavor, but for a large percentage of doctors *they know very little when it comes to nutrition, being fit or losing weight.* And as mentioned, the proof of their advice should be in the pudding. *Do they take their own advice?*

Here is my take on this...if an overweight doctor (or anyone else) is offering weight loss advice, *then why isn't it working for them?* Would you listen to someone tell you how to quit smoking cigarettes if they are still smoking?

My advice is to be careful when someone offers you any advice when it comes to losing weight, especially when the person telling you is carrying a lot of extra weight. My question again is why isn't this advice working for them? Again, let the proof be in the pudding.

I have no issues with doctors *(especially if I broke an arm),* but if the doctor is not following his or her own advice, then I would be cautious on the advice that they may offer you in the area of nutrition or weight loss.

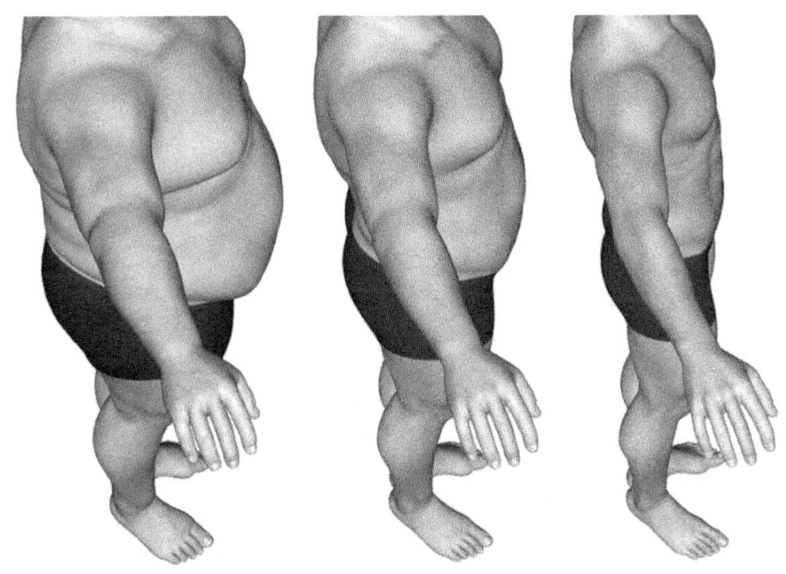

Tip #10
Body fat is STORED ENERGY
begging to be used

Have you ever wondered exactly why the fat on your body is just sitting there? Seriously. What is its purpose?

Here is the deal... *fat is nothing more than STORED ENERGY waiting to be used.* That is it in a nutshell.

But here is the problem... *most people never tap into this body fat* (or stored energy) and here is the reason why:

Most overweight people are always eating foods that keep their insulin high (sorry sugar and processed foods).

In other words, the only way to burn that fat around your belly as a daily energy source (and lose it) is to learn to keep your insulin low throughout the day. Nothing more and nothing less.

Let me say that again...*the only time that you can burn or use the fat around your belly as energy is when your insulin is low.* Use this body fat as your daily energy source and it will eventually disappear.

No ifs, ands, or buts about it.

Understand this important point:

When you eat "manufactured in a factory" food your insulin spikes up and does its job by depositing all of that converted sugar into fat cells. This is the job of insulin and without it we would all die.

Eventually our bellies and hips begin to expand with all of this extra stored fat *that would really love to be burned up if you only allowed it to be used for energy.*

The problem is that we continue to stuff ourselves with high insulin spiking foods *(think pastas, breads, corn, potatoes, junk food, etc.)* that not only convert into fat cells, but more importantly keep our insulin high. This in turn promotes chronic diseases and keeps fat on the body.

Eat pasta, bread, potatoes and cereal, and insulin instantly shoots up and stores as fat cells around your hips. But eat something like a steak and broccoli and it will do just the opposite *since this type of REAL FOOD keeps your insulin low.*

You need to understand that REAL FOOD does not spike your insulin. This is the reason that you can then use body fat as energy, and eventually lose that fat around your belly and hips.

The bottom line... you can only burn that fat around your waistline when your insulin is at a low state. This is why intermittent fasting *(just Google it)* and eating REAL FOOD that keeps your insulin low is the major key to becoming a leaner person.

Choose REAL FOOD, implement intermittent fasting by simply skipping breakfast, and trust me when I say that the fat on your body will now be able to be used as your daily energy source.

Just be ready to go shopping as you will soon need a new wardrobe with all of that body fat being used as energy!

"You need to understand that REAL FOOD does not spike your insulin. This is the reason that you can then use body fat as energy, and eventually lose that fat around your belly and hips."

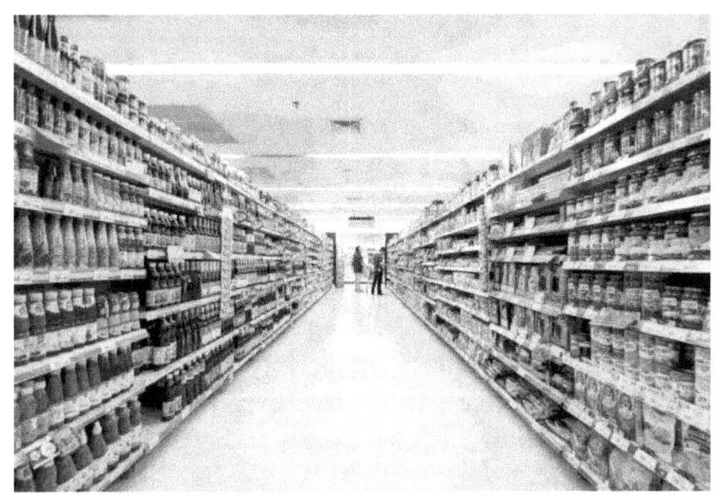

Tip #11
19 store products I would never buy

Following are products that I happened to notice at the grocery store recently and thought I would share what I would never waste my money on:

#1 Sugar Coated Vitamins

We as a nation have become so addicted to sugar that we now have to lace our vitamins *with cancer-feeding sugar*. Wow.

#2 Medications Galore

Hippocrates said *"Let food be thy medicine and medicine be thy food."*

I personally try to avoid all of this stuff as much as possible. In my opinion it is all a bandage to what the real issue is...and that is the *terrible for your health* processed food that is being deposited into your belly every day.

#3 Slim Fast Along With Other Similar Products

Honestly, if Laura Ingalls from the TV series *Little House on the*

Prairie cannot recognize it as being food, then trust me when I say it is not real food.

Please do not waste your time with these types of diet gimmicks. Simply learn to eat REAL FOOD and your hips and belly will begin to shrink.

#4 Joint Juice, etc.

Instead of wasting your money on these types of new products that continually flood the market, try divorcing all sugars and refined carbs *(processed foods)* for one month and see if your joint pain slowly disappears.

Remember if your joints are getting sore then maybe it is telling you to stop putting garbage food into your body.

#5 Orange Juice (and any other juice)

Trust me when I say that all juices are highly concentrated (even 100%) and is recognized as nothing more that sugar when it goes down the hatch.

Insulin instantly shoots up and your body goes into a weird state of shock gulping all of this concentrated stuff down. You can get your Vitamin C from much healthier alternatives.

If you absolutely need your juice fix then simply eat an orange since you will get the fiber with it, and it will not be so highly concentrated.

#6 Sugar Laced Yogurt

Of all the products on the market that totally deceives those who are trying to lose weight, none is more deceptive than the sugar laced dessert called yogurt.

So many consumers have no idea that all of these popular yogurt brands are poor for your health with the added sugar in each little container.

Stay far away from these manufactured desserts. I personally do not care if the label says it is healthy and has only 100 calories. If you want to get rid of that spare tire around your waist, then avoid these deceptive yogurt brands at all cost.

If you must eat yogurt then simply get 100% pure yogurt and throw a few real berries into the container.

#7 All Soda Pops

In my opinion soda pop has to go down as the worst invention that continues to make people overweight. It is basically sugar, carbonated water, and sticky favored syrup.

Listen carefully. *If you are addicted to soda pop, it is really your addiction to sugar.* Take away all of the added sugar and soda pop would sit on the grocery store shelves.

Also, stay away from diet soda pop unless you love to feed your body poison. Artificial sweeteners are as bad or worst than sugar in my opinion.

#8 Processed Boxed Food

The MAJORITY of anything in a box with a label slapped on it saying *food* is a joke in my opinion. Most of this stuff is made in a dirty basement somewhere in New York City. The sad reality is that most people *will basically eat anything as long as it is classified as a food product.*

Just stay away from this garbage unless you want to stay or continue to get fat. Most of these processed foods have very little nutritional value.

#9 Bottled Tea/Lemonade Products

Whenever I see a person buying these tea or lemonade bottled products, I instantly think of all of the sugar that they are putting into their bodies. Trust me when I say they are going to eventually get fat drinking this stuff.

These types of tea and lemonade products are nothing more than sugar water with tea flavoring. Stay with unsweetened tea as the safe alternative.

#10 Starbucks Bottled Drinks

31 grams of sugar *(over 7 teaspoons of sugar)* in one bottle and people still buy this stuff? The only thing I can say on products like these is if you want a bigger belly or more fat on your body, then this should be your go-to drink.

#11 Captain Crunch and His Cohorts...

Instead of Tony the Tiger saying "THEEEEEIIIIIR GREAT", he should say "THEEEEEIIIIIR FATTENING!"

Stop being deceived into believing that these boxed cereals are innocent with their colorful and cute characters peddling this unhealthy sugar loaded stuff.

The cereal business is a billion dollar a year industry and is here to stay. *They will also continue to brain wash your children with the cute cartoon commercials that convey that their cereal is innocent and fun to eat.*

I look at the whole aisle of these colorful cereal boxes at my friendly grocery store and see nothing more than cancer causing sugar transporters.

Listen carefully. Boxed cereal will pack on the pounds with all of the sugar and refined carbs in each spoonful. *I personally would call it a morning dessert.*

#12 Granola Bars

Do not be deceived with the healthy packaging that they come in. The vast majority of these bars are simply glorified candy bars and will give you brain fog with the hidden sugar and loaded carbs in each bar.

#13 Skinny Pop Popcorn, Veggie Straws, and All of the Other

Chips in a Bag...

Trust me when I say that Skinny Pop Popcorn will not make you skinny. *Remember also that they feed corn to cows to make them fat.*

All of these bagged snack products give naive consumers the impression that they are healthy, when in reality they will eventually make you fat.

Bottom line... Stay away from all of these bagged snack products if you want to get your high school weight back.

#14 Candy, Candy, Candy

Bottom line on eating any form of candy or candy bar:

It is just a sugar fix that you crave and nothing more. The real reason that people love their candy or candy bar is because of the high percentage of sugar in each bite.

The sad truth is that a majority of people within our society are addicted to sugar and are totally clueless to this fact. *Sugar makes you fat, PERIOD.*

#15 Alcohol

Outside of the fact that I personally have zero desire for any form of alcohol, drinking any form of alcohol converts to sugar in your body, spikes up the insulin *(a really bad thing),* and will eventually give you a spare tire around the waistline.

#16 Clear Bottled Cooking Oils

If you want to restore your health, then you need to get these types of cooking oils *(Vegetable Oil, Corn Oil, Canola Oil, etc.)* out of your kitchen. Use either Olive Oil or Coconut Oil instead.

Also, my advice is to never buy anything at a restaurant that is cooked in oil *(sorry french fry lovers)* as you will be putting this unhealthy oil into your body. Avoid these cooking oils and your belly will begin to shrink.

#17 Store Brought and Restaurant Bread

If you are looking to expand your waistline, my recommendation is to eat store bought breads. Restaurant bread is also included as well *(sorry Panera Bread)*.

Please do not be fooled by the skinny happy people in the TV commercials telling you how healthy their bread is. *If they were honest they would have overweight actors and actresses in these commercials peddling their fat producing bread.*

#18 Honey Buns and All Other Bakery Fat Foods

If you are interested in expanding your waistline, then these types of products should also be your go-to foods.

And guess what? Trans fats are also included in these products at no extra charge!

#19 The Standard American Diet (SAD Diet) Fast Food Market

This final one is really going to hurt some of you, and the sad fact is that the vast majority of overweight people in our great nation live off of this food weekly.

That is a major reason that we live in a serious fat nation. I have said this before and will say it again...

If Laura Ingalls from Little House on the Prairie cannot recognize it as a food product, then trust me with I say that it is not REAL FOOD.

If you want to get back your younger and healthier body weight, my recommendation is to avoid all fast food restaurants as much as possible.

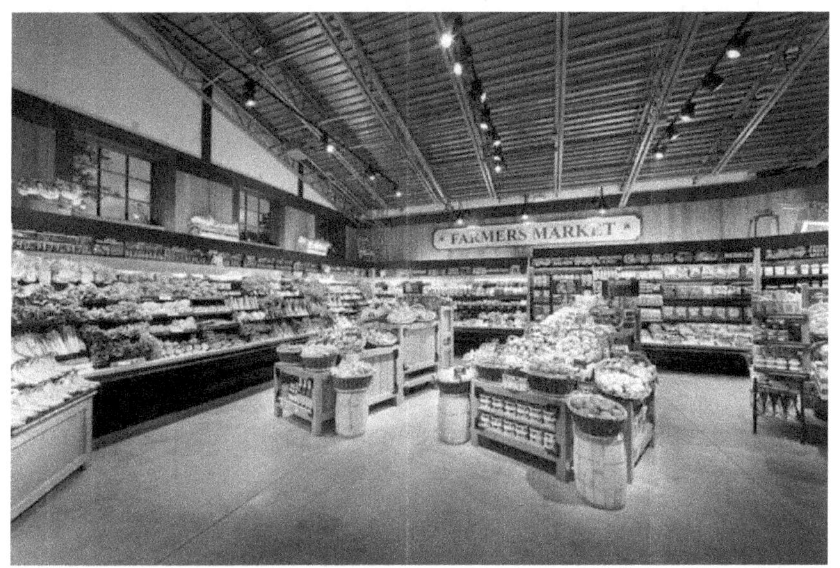

Tip #12
19 Store Products I WOULD BUY

In the last chapter I mentioned 19 unhealthy grocery store products I would never buy. In this chapter I would like to share 19 grocery store products that I would buy to lose weight and become healthier.

So if you are serious about feeling better and losing weight, here are 19 *products I would have no problem buying if I wanted to lose 10, 20, 50, or 100+ pounds:*

#1 Real Cheese

Don't be afraid of eating cheese if your body agrees with it. Having it in moderation is not a problem. Just make sure to avoid any processed cheese *(think Kraft wrapped slices or Velveeta)* as these types of processed foods are bad for your health.

#2 Veggies

It's a no-brainer. I personally would not eat potatoes since our bodies recognize it as a lump of sugar and will instantly spike up the insulin *(which will keep fat on the body by making you burn sugar and carbs instead of body fat).*

#3 Some Fruit

To be truthful I stay primarily with berries (blue, black) since the majority of fruit will shoot up your insulin as it converts to sugar, and this is not a good thing if you are trying to become lean. *Keep your insulin low and you will lose weight.*

If your goal is to either get healthier or lose weight my recommendation is to keep fruit to a bare minimum *due to the effect that it has on spiking the insulin.* Eat foods that keep your insulin low and you will become healthier and get leaner.

#4 Frozen Beef

Just make sure that it is 100% beef since some of these frozen hamburger products actually put fillers into the beef. Unbelievable but true.

Buying fresh beef is obviously the best choice, but having frozen on hand when you do not have any fresh beef fills the gap in moments like these.

#5 100% Natural Peanut Butter

A great treat in moderation and having a spoonful every now and then is perfectly fine as it will keep your insulin low. *It also fills the gap for those with a sweet tooth.*

I use it with my coconut fat bombs *(just Google it),* and peanut butter is a great treat once you totally eliminate sugar from your life.

Also, remember to only buy the 100% Natural Peanut Butter as all of the others have added additional ingredients which in my opinion totally ruin the natural flavor.

#6 Meats (Steaks & Hamburger)

If you are serious about losing weight *(and are not a vegan),* then I highly recommend eating meat. I personally eat it almost every day and recommend *Chuck Eye Steak* as it tastes great and has a lot of excellent fat on it. These steaks are similar to a Ribeye steak but at a lower cost, and will totally satisfy your hunger.

For hamburgers I recommend the burgers with the most fat (73% / 27%) as these are the juiciest and best tasting.

If you are still afraid of eating fats then it sounds like you are still stuck in the science of the 1960's *(just Google it to get reeducated on this subject).* These fats are perfectly safe and will help you to lose that belly fat by maintaining low insulin and keeping you full for a very long time.

#7 Canned Veggies

Yes, I do understand that getting vegetables fresh is the best thing, but there will be times when you may not have any at home.

This will be the perfect time to have canned veggies that will work for moments like these.

#8 Chicken (with the skin left on)

Please stop being afraid of chicken skin as it will not make you fat. If you really want to treat yourself, *then fry the chicken in good old fashioned lard with the skin left on.*

It tastes seriously great *(like grandma use to make).* And please stop being deceived by the government's recommendation that you should use vegetable oil or a myriad of other processed oils instead. *These products are terrible for your health!*

Remember that big government's primary interest is in keeping America hooked on these *very profitable* corporate cooking oils. Trust me when I say that every one of these will eventually damage your body.

#9 Fish / Salmon

You cannot go wrong with adding fish to your diet. Just stay away from all of those breaded fish in a box. Stay with fresh fish if at all possible.

#10 Bacon *(yes, bacon)*

There was a time that I rarely if ever ate bacon as I thought it would clog my arteries, raise my cholesterol, and give me a heart attack. *Of course that was when I was uneducated and still living in the science of the 1960's.*

I personally like to get the thickest bacon, and recommend buying it without nitrates if at all possible.

If you want to lose weight, then make sure to add bacon to your diet. *Also be sure to throw away all of those terrible boxed processed diet foods that really are unhealthy for you.*

#11 Frozen Veggies

Frozen veggies are great when you do not have fresh veggies available for a meal. Just steam them and throw a mixture of 100% melted butter and coconut oil on the veggies for a serious great tasting dish.

Eat this way and you will lose weight.

#12 100% REAL Butter

Whenever I see a person in line at the grocery store buying margarine or a tub of *I Can't Believe it's Not Butter,* I think to myself that they have zero clue on how much damage they are doing to their body.

My other impression is that they will have some serious health issues down the road consuming these types of products.

My advice is to only use 100% REAL BUTTER. All of the other fake products in the butter section are terrible for your health.

If you are serious about losing weight and restoring your health to the maximum, then stick with 100% real butter. *It's healthy and no it will not give you a heart attack, clog your arteries, or make your fat.*

Eat butter and you will lose weight.

#13 Eggs

Please do not listen to the government when it comes to eggs. They are perfectly safe.

#14 Sour Cream

I personally love all of the fat in sour cream as it is satisfying and will keep a body lean.

My only advice is to avoid at all costs any food product that says *low fat* or *no fat* as they take out the good fat and replace it with unhealthy additives (sugar being one of them).

So remember that if you want to lose weight, never buy anything that says *low fat* or *no fat*. If you really want to lose weight, then let healthy fats be an important part of your daily diet.

#15 Water

I just wish I would have patented this idea years ago. I mean who would have thought that one day we would buy water from a bottle?

But seriously, *99.9% of any liquid drink in a can or bottle is terrible for your health* (think soda pop, juices, energy drinks, and the dozens of other bottled or canned beverage on the market).

Compared to all of the other drink choices out there, water is by far your best choice.

#16 Coconut Oil

I am sold on this stuff and recommend putting it in your body everyday for some serious great health benefits. *Of all of the health products out there, buying coconut oil is my #1 recommendation.*

Simply Google the benefits of this amazing oil as they are too many to list here. If you want to feel better and get rid of brain fog, then I would highly recommend consuming coconut oil daily in order to get healthy fats into your body and brain.

Your brain is made primarily of fat and coconut oil will do wonders in helping it function at its best throughout the day.

#17 Olive Oil

Please go into your kitchen and throw away AS FAST AS YOU CAN all of the clear bottled cooking oils that you have wasted your money on *(think Crisco, Vegetable oil, Canola oil, Corn oil, etc)*.

If you absolutely need to use cooking oil, then my four choices would be olive oil, coconut oil, lard, and butter. I personally rarely ever fry anything, but the above would be my choice.

#18 Avocados

Avocados are a serious great source of fat *(comparable with coconut oil)* and outstanding for your health.

#19 Broccoli

Since broccoli is my favorite vegetable I had to throw it into my list. It is an amazing product and will do wonders for your overall health. I personally try to eat it at almost every meal!

If you really want a great broccoli dish be sure to melt coconut oil and butter on top of it. *I am quite confident that if you give it a try you too will fall in love with this powerful and seriously healthy vegetable.*

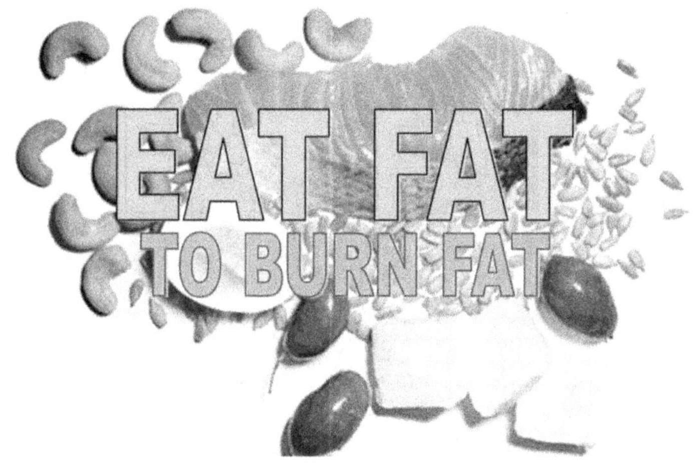

Tip #13
Make fats your friend if you want to lose weight

One of the major reasons that you cannot lose weight is because *you cannot grasp the truth that eating healthy fats will eventually put you on the road to getting leaner.*

It is time to get over your fear of fat if you want to get back the weight that you once had in those earlier years when you were trimmer.

One of the major reasons that you have gained all of that weight is because *you have listened to the government and so-called health experts over the years tell you not to eat fat.* They were wrong and continue to be wrong.

Listen carefully... your body needs healthy fats, and NO *they do not clog your arteries, raise your cholesterol, give you a heart attack, or make you fat. Never has and never will.*

The real enemy to the above diseases is sugar, fake cooking oils, processed foods, and trans fats. Healthy fats do not do this.

Throw away your Crisco and vegetable oil and replace them with coconut oil or olive oil if you want to lose weight and become healthy again.

I personally try to live daily off of *70% healthy fats, 25% protein, and 5% carbs,* and cannot tell you how healthy I feel every day now that I eat good fats.

I try to eat a lot of healthy fats daily and it has not added an ounce of fat to my body... *never has and never will.*

Healthy fats are not dangerous for you. It is a flawed fable that most of America still believes, and a major reason that we as a nation are overweight. *Simply ditch the bad carbs, replace them with healthy fats, and you will become leaner.*

Give healthy fats a try for one month *and divorce your high sugar and carb diet.* Not only will you become healthier and think clearer, but your pant size will continue to go down. If you are going to eat carbs, then remember to only stick with healthy carbs *(think veggies).*

The real culprit to poor health is Crisco and bottle of vegetable oil sitting in your kitchen, along with all of those processed food products in your cupboards. Again, throw it all away and replace it with eating healthy fats if you want to be lean again!

Stop listening to your overweight doctor or the debunked science of the 1960's and reeducate yourself on making your daily food intake a high percentage of healthy fats. *Your body and brain will thank you for it.*

Start making coconut oil, eggs, animal fat *(think juicy steaks & bacon),* healthy vegetables, and avocados a good part of your diet, and you will begin to see your belly and hips disappear.

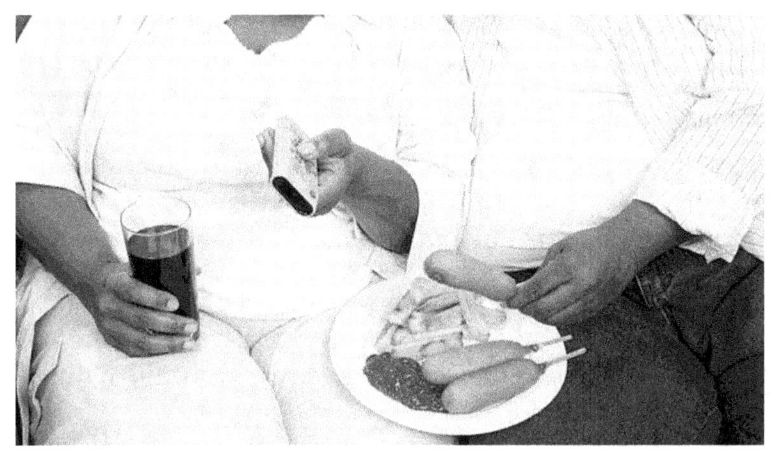

Tip #14
Why are most people over 40 overweight?

A couple of years ago I was waiting at an airport and noticed a very rare occurrence that is seldom seen in our day and age.

The airport was crowded and there was a pilot standing near where I was sitting that looked in his mid fifties. What caught my attention was the fact that this pilot was seriously fit.

He looked super healthy and lean. Unlike the vast majority of men around him who were overweight and had the typical big belly, this guy totally stood out as someone who understands how to eat right. *My only regret was that I did not go up and ask him about his diet.*

So why do we seldom see a person over 40 (or is it 30?) who is not overweight? Statistics state that 67% of our nation is overweight and 1 out of 3 people are obese. *There clearly is a problem happening within our food-is-everywhere society.*

So here is my two cents on why most people over 40 are overweight:

It is simply the years (and decades) of eating terrible food, period. Nothing more, and nothing less.

Please stop believing that with age automatically comes a big belly or big hips. This is not normal and *our bodies were never designed to carry all of that extra weight around.*

Being overweight is one major reason why we have so many chronic diseases along with getting new replacement parts on our body. Our bodies eventually break down with all of the extra weight that it is forced to carry.

You really do not have to stay fat for the rest of your life. The real culprit to your overweight body is the terrible selection of food that you have been putting into your belly for decades, and the result is clearly seen in the mirror.

You alone will make the final choice in whether you want to stay fat for the rest of your life. But I can guarantee that if you completely do a 180 degree turn and totally change your eating habits, *weight will begin to fall off of your body.*

Listen, there is a fit and lean person within you waiting to get out if you will simply stop feeding your body all of that processed food and start to eat REAL FOOD instead *(like 'ol Abe Lincoln would have eaten).*

We live in *an unhealthy food culture* where most people are continually stuffing themselves with manufactured food *(mostly processed)*. My advice is to stop feeding yourself this fat producing food, and only eat when you are actually hungry.

This is the way we were designed to eat. Simply learn to listen to your body as it will tell you when it is truly hungry.

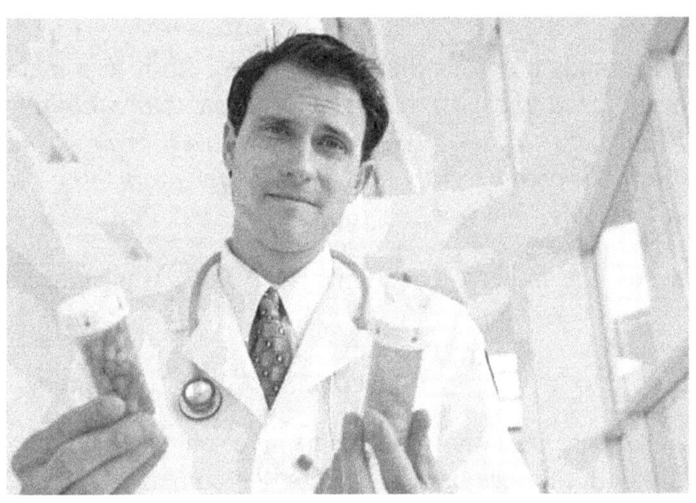

Tip #15
Why I do not trust the majority of doctors

I really do not get it on why so many people *put their complete trust in their doctor in regards to health and nutrition.*

It also boggles my brain that so many people will never question why their doctor continually pushes hard to pronounce prescription drugs to take without batting an eye.

Personally I don't get it. Why in the world would you trust a doctor who continually offers drugs for what ails you? Also, most doctors never will ask a patient about their diet. *To me this clearly displays an incompetent person who really is not qualified to help others in the area of health and nutrition.*

Listen, it is the food that you are feeding your body all of these years that should be addressed by doctors. Pills are simply bandages and does nothing more than mask the real problem, which in my opinion is a poor diet.

Sure there are a few holistic sound doctors out there who get it and truly understands how our diet is the main culprit to a majority of our illnesses, *but the vast majority of doctors are nothing more than pill pushers to the masses who have been brainwashed with the 100's of TV commercials they have watched pushing the latest and greatest drug for what ails you.*

Hippocrates, the father of medicine, 431 B.C., was right when he said:

"Let food be thy medicine and medicine be thy food."

We as humans were not meant to live on prescription drugs, especially with the serious side effects that come with them.

I personally would find a doctor who not only takes care of himself, but who really understands nutrition and how food plays a major role in how healthy we are. *Why would I want to listen to an unhealthy drug pushing doctor in regards to my health?*

In my opinion, if a doctor is happy-go-lucky when it comes to passing out pills, I would personally find someone else who will get to the root of the majority of health issues... *and that is a poor diet.*

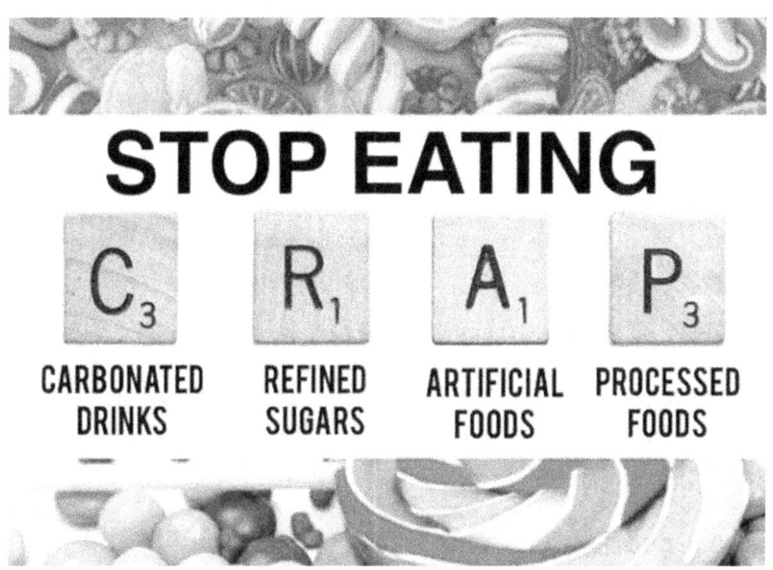

Tip #16
4 items in your kitchen that I recommend throwing away

Here are 4 items in your kitchen that will eventually do some serious damage to your body. I'll also give you a replacement to each of these items that would be a much better healthy choice:

#1 THROW AWAY ALL FAKE BUTTERS

This includes all types of margarines and *I Can't Believe It's Not Butter*. Ignore what our caring government nutritionist experts say as these fake butters are terrible for your health.

Replace all of the above with *REAL 100% Butter* if you want to be healthy. And no, it will not clog your arteries, give you a heart attack, or make you fat.

#2 ALL FAKE COOKING OILS

Products like Crisco, vegetable oil, canola oil, and the rest of those clear oil bottles that line your friendly grocery store shelves are nothing more than poison to your body, and in my opinion is the real culprit to heart disease and overall bad health.

Replace all of the above *with coconut oil, olive oil, 100% butter, or good old fashion lard* if you want to become healthier or lose weight.

#3 CAPTAIN CRUNCH AND HIS SUGARY FRIENDS

It is ridiculous that all of these cereals proudly proclaim all of the added vitamins that are included on the front of the box.

Listen, the majority of these cereals is nothing more than sugar-laced morning desserts and should be avoided if you want to restore your health.

If you absolutely must eat breakfast *(which I do not recommend...just Google Intermittent Fasting),* then eat foods that will not shoot up your insulin (which will store then fat). Eggs and bacon are a great replacement if you want to become lean.

#4 BEVERAGES IN A CAN OR BOTTLE

The majority of drinking products in a can or bottle will not only make you unhealthy, but will give you a spare tire around the waistline. This includes soda pop, juices (even 100%), and the dozens of other beverages found in a fancy can *(sorry cola lovers).*

Replace all of these with a product called water if you want to get that high school weight back again.

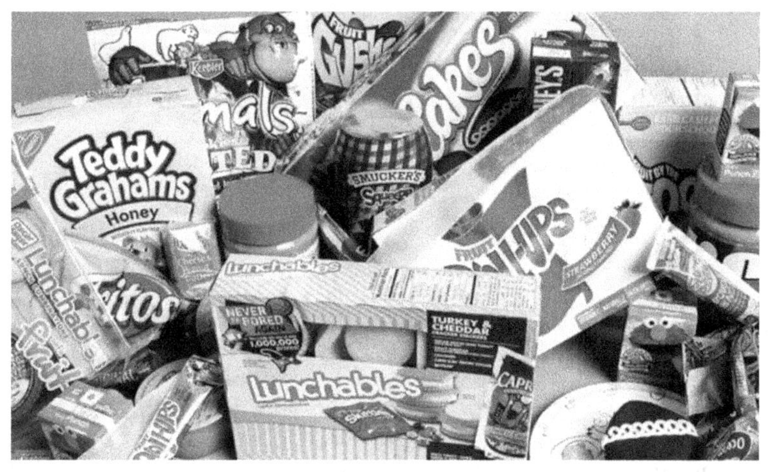

Tip #17
The 3 main reasons that you overeat

For many people having years or decades of a weight problem is a result of overeating food products that are unhealthy (think processed foods).

Here are the 3 main reasons that you may overeat:

#1 YOU MAY OVEREAT BECAUSE THERE IS AN ABUNDANCE OF CHEAP FOOD AVAILABLE.

There has never been a time in history where a society has had such an abundance of cheap and unhealthy food available.

In my opinion the majority of food that is available at the local grocery store or restaurant is unhealthy for us, *but highly profitable for the companies and restaurants that are offering them.*

The first reason that you may overeat is because of this over-abundance of food on every other street corner. It seems that a large percentage of overweight people simply are not disciplined enough to stop consuming all of this cheap and available food.

Commercial after commercial tempts us to run out and buy a

greasy chicken leg from KFC, or run to the store and purchase a cheap and unhealthy frozen pizza. With so much cheap food available, we have become a fat and undisciplined nation.

#2 YOU MAY OVEREAT BECAUSE OF THE COMFORT THAT FOOD BRINGS.

The second reason that many people overeat is because stuffing their belly is a habitual way of being comforted. It may be that they came from a dysfunctional home and learned early on that stuffing their belly was an escape from any early emotional pain.

To some people food is a comforting drug and allows them temporary relief from any hurts that may have occurred in the past.

Remember that when you were younger you did not have the mature cognitive thinking to deal with dysfunction within your home, *so your drug of choice may have become food.*

But now that you are older, you now have more intelligence to deal with past pains. In other words, you are more emotionally mature to work through any pains from the past without having to run to the refrigerator every time you begin thinking about past hurts.

#3 A PERSON OVEREATS BECAUSE BAD FOODS MESSES UP LEPTIN (which tells your brain that you are full).

Scientists have now discovered a hormone called Leptin. The job of Leptin is to tell your brain that you have had enough to eat.

The problem is that junk food and sugar interferes with Leptin doing its job, and your brain then has a hard time recognizing Leptin so you stay hungry longer.

This then causes a problem with your pancreas which produces insulin to help regulate sugar in your system.

The more sugar in your bloodstream, the harder your pancreas has to work. And remember, an overworked pancreas will eventually bring either obesity, type 2 diabetes, metabolic syndrome, heart disease, or liver disease.

So what do I recommend if you have an overeating issue in your personal life?

#1 Eat only when you are absolutely hungry *(divorce it as a recreational activity)*.

#2 Stop using eating as an emotional comfort pill. You now are more mature and can deal with past hurts with a more heightened degree of intelligence. There are now better ways to deal with past hurts than simply stuffing yourself with unhealthy food.

#3 Let the hormone Leptin work for you in telling your brain that you are full *by not letting sugar and junk food destroy the communication between the hormone Leptin and your brain.*

"The first reason that you overeat is because of this over-abundance of food on every other street corner."

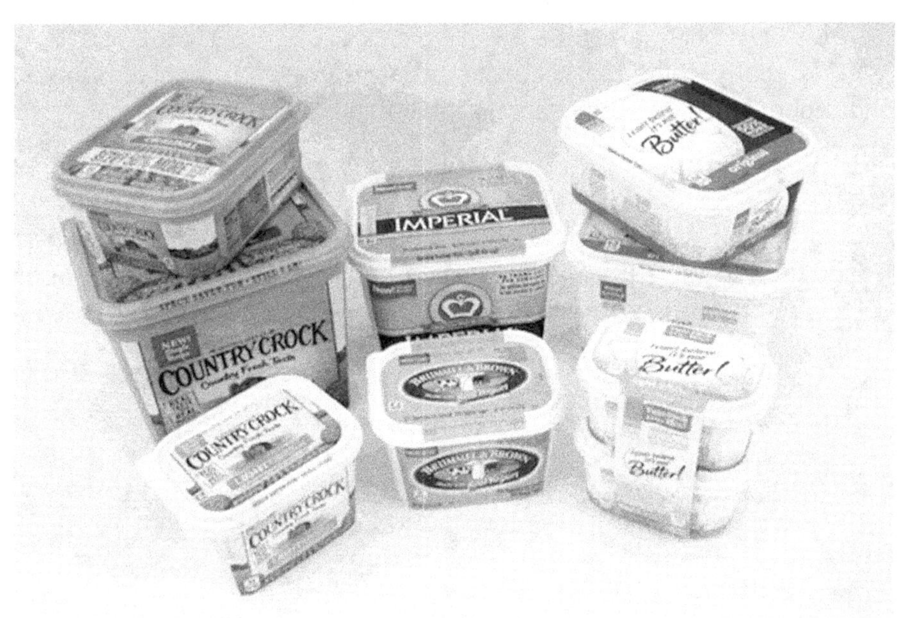

Tip #18
3 signs that identify a person is clueless to being healthy

Here are 3 quick signs that can easily identify someone who has very little concept on how to be healthy:

1. They still use margarine

If you see a person who still uses margarine they are clueless as this is poison. *Margarine is but one molecule away from being PLASTIC, and shares 27 ingredients with PAINT.* Stay with 100% pure butter instead.

2. They still think animal fat will clog their arteries, raise their cholesterol, give them a heart attack, or make them fat.

People who still believe this silly statement are stuck in the science of the 1960's and need reeducation. My recommendation is to go to Google and learn about the clear benefits of healthy fats.

It is really your daily consumption of sugar, processed foods, refined carbs, and trans fats that will make a person sick and fat.

3. They say sugar is not toxic to your body

The reason most people won't believe this is because they are addicted to the stuff and don't even know it. *In my opinion, sugar is and always will be the #1 culprit to our health and obesity epidemic.*

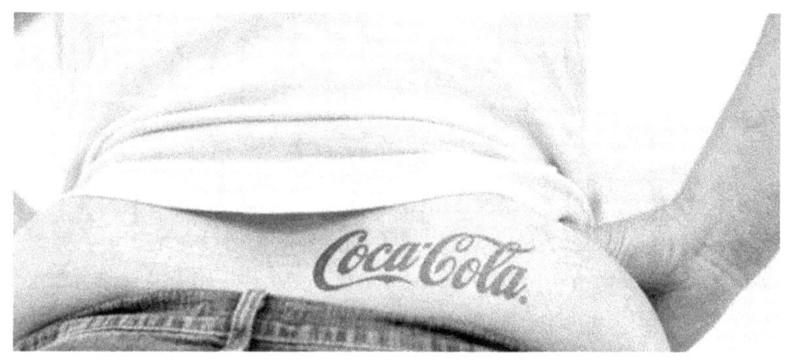

Tip #19
Sugar has made you fat, period

Did you know that there are 61 names for sugar and that it is in approximately 80% of all grocery store items?

No matter what label that it is given *(call it brown sugar, agave nectar, coconut sugar, high fructose corn syrup, honey)*, all of it is the #1 reason that the majority of people in any given crowd are fat

Listen, *sugar is sugar is sugar is sugar.* Please don't be fooled into thinking that something like agave nectar is a healthy alternative just because it happens to be sold at your local health food store. It will raise your insulin and store fat on your body.

All of these 61 sugar names enter your system and immediately raise your insulin. This is a major reason that you have a spare tire around your waist. *Simply quit sugar and you will eventually see that tire disappear.*

I always laugh inside whenever I hear of a person completing a *"7 day sugar fast"* or a *"30 day sugar detox"* and then going back to this fat producing poison.

I have also noticed that each person who completes one of these challenges also tells everyone how much more alert and energized they feel by getting off of this legal and addictive drug.

They also proclaim that they had lost 5, 7, or 10 pounds simply by getting off of sugar. They cannot praise their absence away from this poison enough.

But the part that makes me laugh and scratch my head is *why in the world do they finish their successful dry sugar challenge and then go back to consuming this unhealthy product?* They go back to a daily diet of sugar, and then brain fog and weight gain eventually return.

Bottom line... I have come to the conclusion that the majority of overweight people are addicted to sugar and processed foods *(which convert to sugar),* and simply refuse to quit this fat producing substance.

Either continue your love affair with sugar and stay overweight, or say goodbye to this toxin, and become a leaner and healthier person... you alone make that choice.

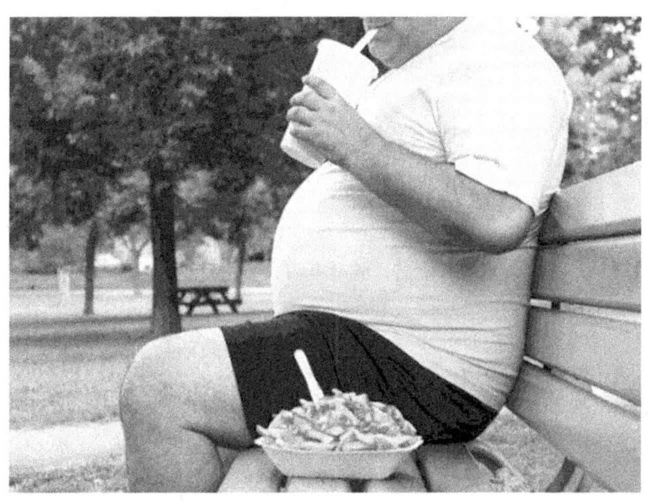

Tip #20
Does anyone honestly enjoy being fat?

There is a movement today in our media that overweight people should love and embrace their fatness and accept how they look.

I personally have no issue with this and agree that we need to accept ourselves for who we are. Each of us individually is unique in our own special way. I get it.

But that is not what I want to talk about. I want to focus on the serious and crippling health issues that comes with being overweight.

The real issue about being overweight that I want to target is that *it is bad for your health,* and is a doorway to so many serious chronic diseases. Every health expert agrees with this. So here is my point:

It is not the issue of being overweight. What is the issue is how damaging being overweight can be to both your health and daily lifestyle.

So here is my question again:

Do you honestly DEEP DOWN INSIDE want to be overweight?

I mean if you had the choice to instantly drop that 20 or 40 or 100+ extra pounds, would you do it in a heartbeat?

My personal thought is that the majority (if not all) who are overweight would instantly scream YES to the above question without hesitation.

Let me get to the point... You do not have to stay overweight and I am here to tell you that *there is a leaner person inside of you waiting to come out.*

I personally do not care if you have always been *the fat guy or fat girl in the room* all of your life. You CAN DO THIS and lose the weight.

You and you alone can change, *but it is your choice alone.* Nobody can do this for you. Yes it takes courage and the odds are stacked against you, especially as you look back at all of the dieting failures that have occurred in your past attempts.

But I stand here and with a sincere heart want to tell you that you can lose all of that weight that you have been carrying around for years if you simply do the following three things:

1. *Divorce Sugar (weight will instantly start dropping).*

2. *Eat REAL FOOD (If 'ol Abe Lincoln did not eat it neither should you...processed foods are keeping you overweight).*

3. *Intermittent Fasting (just stop eating breakfast).*

These above 3 tips are super healthy for your body, and within a week you will begin to notice a serious difference in how you feel.

Make the above 3 tips your new lifestyle, and not only will you feel better and have a clearer mind, but that leaner person inside of you will soon become the new you.

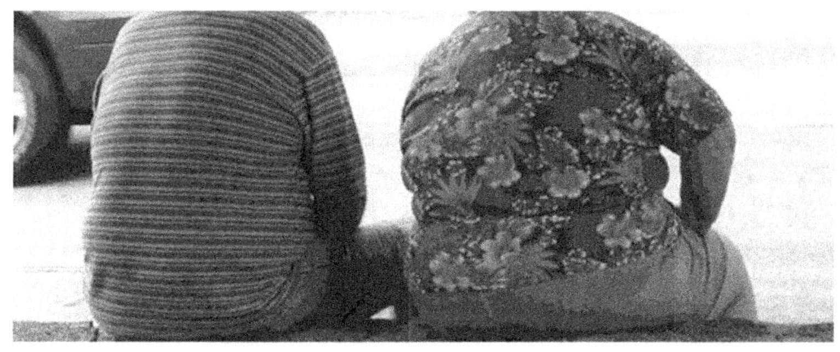

Tip #21
Why do so many people gain back their weight?

Why is it that a high percentage of people who succeed in losing weight always seem to put it back on?

We all know those who were very successful in dropping a lot of weight, and then for some unknown reason they eventually put the weight back on.

Let me offer you the 3 main reasons why this happens:

#1 PEOPLE GAIN BACK THEIR WEIGHT BECAUSE THEY FOLLOWED A SILLY CALORIE RESTRICTING DIET

I have said this often and will say it again...

Calorie restricting diets eventually fail because we as humans eventually get tired of always feeling hungry and restricted.

It is the same old song and dance for the majority of dieters who follow one of these calorie restricting diets. They begin losing weight and after a few months get tired of always feeling restricted.

My advice is to throw away calorie counting altogether and cut sugar and processed foods completely out of your life. Now begin to eat REAL FOOD if you want to permanently lose weight.

#2 PEOPLE GAIN BACK THEIR WEIGHT BECAUSE THEY CANNOT LET GO OF A SECRET SUGAR ADDICTION

As mentioned in previous chapters, if you want to permanently lose weight, then sugar has to be kicked out of your life. *There are no ifs, ands, or buts about it.*

And yes I understand that sugar has been a big part of your life for decades (been there and done that), but it is almost impossible to maintain a healthy weight if you continue to court sugar.

Remember also that when we make a conscious decision to get completely rid of sugar, we will also begin to stop eating *all of the processed junk foods that line approximately 80% of our friendly grocery store shelves.*

Ridding yourself of all forms of sugar that lace the majority of foods at your grocery store will also open up a new world of learning to eat REAL FOOD instead.

This alone will easily assist you in losing weight by the simple act of divorcing all sugars and processed foods from your life.

#3 PEOPLE GAIN BACK THEIR WEIGHT BECAUSE THEY FEEL UNCOMFORTABLE IN THEIR NEW HEALTHIER BODY

The final reason that people revert back to being overweight is because they have a hard time adjusting to a leaner and healthier version of themselves.

For years *(or decades)* they have viewed themselves as the "fat person" and for some reason cannot come to terms with the new leaner person staring back at them in the mirror.

They also may have a hard time adjusting to the way others may now be treating them *(whether good or bad)* with their new and improved body weight. *Old friends may also have a difficult time adjusting to the new leaner you, and may even start to treat you differently whether they recognize it or not.*

I personally applaud anyone who has permanently kept weight off because it honestly takes courage and determination.

You will definitely be joining a minority since approximately 67% of our adult population is overweight. And it is sad to say, *but there may be a few overweight friends who may become uncomfortable with your new weight loss success.*

My advice is to maintain your courage and follow through on your weight loss goal. *Become a positive example and model for others* by being available to assist and answer questions from those who may want to lose weight as well.

Since you have zero control on how others may react to your weight loss success, *simply love them and remember to offer any helpful advice to anyone who may ask you.*

"My advice is to throw away calorie counting altogether and simply cut sugar completely out of your life. Now begin to eat REAL FOOD if you want to permanently lose weight."

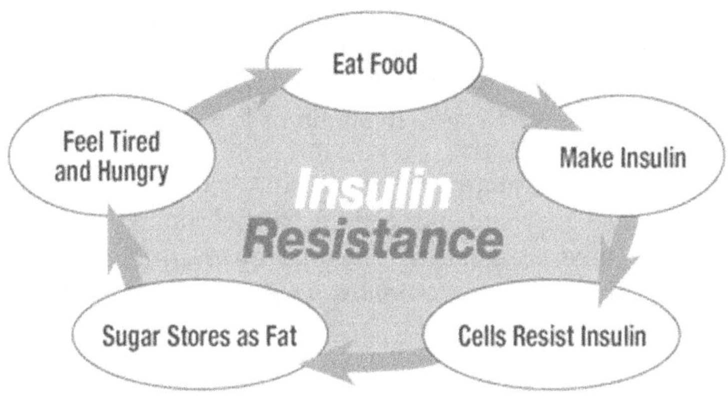

Tip #22
Your weight problem is a hormonal issue

You will hear this often as the key to losing weight, so let me get straight to the point on why I believe the majority of people are overweight:

It is a hormonal issue and having high insulin is what keeps weight on a person. Control your insulin and you will control your weight.

Eating the right foods that keep your insulin low throughout the day is the key to losing weight. This is because when your insulin is low your body is now allowed to go into a fat burning mode which then uses your stored fat as energy *(the healthy way to lose weight)*.

One of the main reasons that most people do not understand this is simply because *there is no money to be made by announcing this fact.*

All of those television diet commercials out there continually make millions selling their unhealthy diet foods, but never tackle the real issue, which is keeping a high insulin state within our body.

This is why it is so important to avoid foods that spike your insulin. The Standard American Diet *(or SAD Diet)* is absolutely terrible for anyone wanting to maintain or lose weight.

Please do not believe those who push a calorie restricting diet simply because they are not getting to the real issue of how to permanently take weight off. *Calorie restricting diets are not sustainable. This is the reason most people eventually quit.*

If you sincerely are tired of carrying those extra pounds around your hips and belly, then I would highly recommend that you learn to eat foods that keep your insulin low *(sorry bread and pasta lovers).*

Do this and I can guarantee that you will soon be burning fat as your daily energy source, and lose weight in the process.

Keep your insulin low with healthy foods and you will *now be allowed to burn your body fat as your daily energy source.* This is how unwanted fat will eventually disappear from your body.

Remember that everything hinges on keeping your insulin level low when it comes to becoming a leaner person, period.

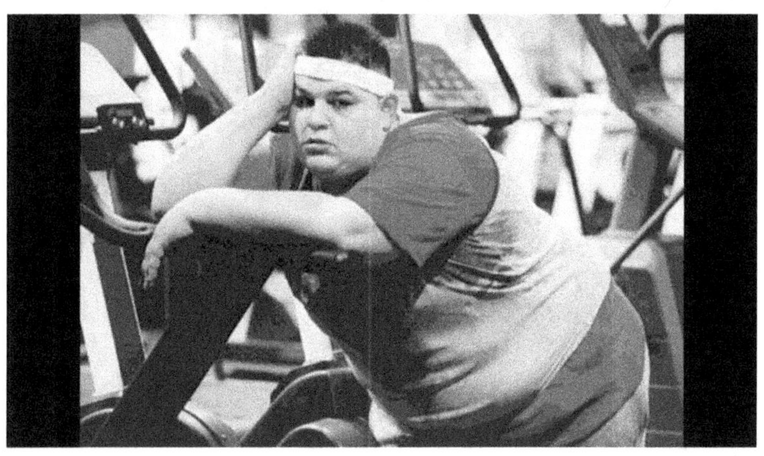

Tip #23
Exercise is not the answer to losing weight

There is a misconception out there that the way to get your belly and hips smaller is to join a gym and exercise. Trust me when I say that weight loss has very little to do with exercise.

Sure exercise has some great benefits, and I would recommend it to anyone. Whether it is going for walks around the neighborhood, taking an aerobics class, or joining a local gym, exercise is outstanding for both mind and body.

But losing weight is not one of those benefits.

Sure you may lose a few pounds sweating on the treadmill, but believing that exercise is the key to weight loss is an incorrect belief.

Here is what you need to understand...

90% of weight loss is done in the kitchen. The only true way that you can permanently keep weight off is by completely changing your diet. Avoid foods that spike your insulin and your body will slowly begin to become leaner.

When you learn to eat foods that keep your insulin low, your body will reward you by letting go of the weight that you so desperately want to get rid of. *Now you are allowing body fat to be burned for your daily energy source.*

My advice is to focus your weight loss program primarily on learning to keep your insulin low throughout the day with intermittent fasting and the right food selections. Do this and your weight will drop.

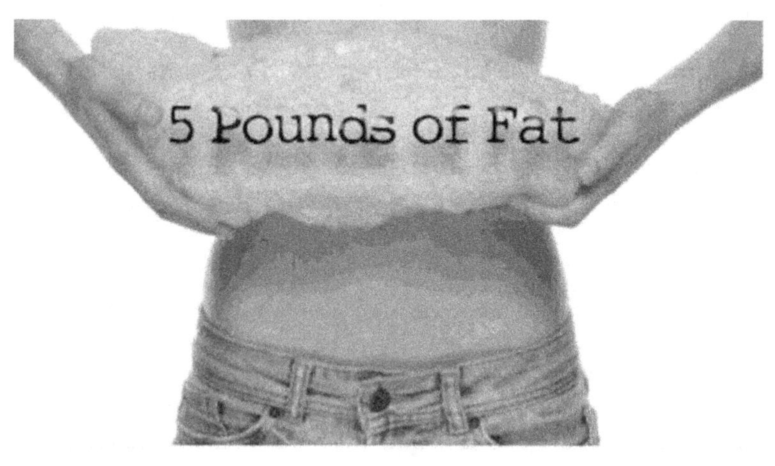

Tip #24
Using body fat as your daily energy source

Fat is a backup source of energy to fuel a person when carbohydrates are not available. This is known as being in *a state of ketosis* and is the key to tapping into your stored fat as a daily energy source.

Ketosis is the state that your body enters into when it starts converting stored fat into ketones to use as fuel for your cells. Do this and body fat starts to disappear.

If you eat sugar and processed foods (carbs), you will never enter into a state of ketosis. Instead, your body will only use all that glucose (sugars and carbs) as a fuel and never use the stored fat on your body.

So what is the key to burning fat as your energy source and essentially losing fat on your body? *The key again is found in the hormone known as insulin.*

The Standard American Diet *(or SAD Diet)* is the perfect storm for a person to store fat on his or her body simply because eating the way that our government promotes keeps our insulin high *(which is a bad thing)*.

This poor recommended diet makes us store fat on the body by promoting high insulin, and also becomes a major gateway to many chronic diseases.

Remember that if your body is in a constant state of high insulin *(through poor food choices)*, it will be almost impossible to burn your body fat as an energy source.

In order to lose weight a person needs to use his or her stored fat *as the primary energy source* throughout the day. And the only way to "tap into" stored fat as your energy source is to keep your insulin low.

Also remember that it is the insulin in your body that ultimately determines whether fat will be used as energy. The simple formula if you would like to lose weight is this:

Keep Insulin Low (by food choices & fasting) = LOSE WEIGHT.

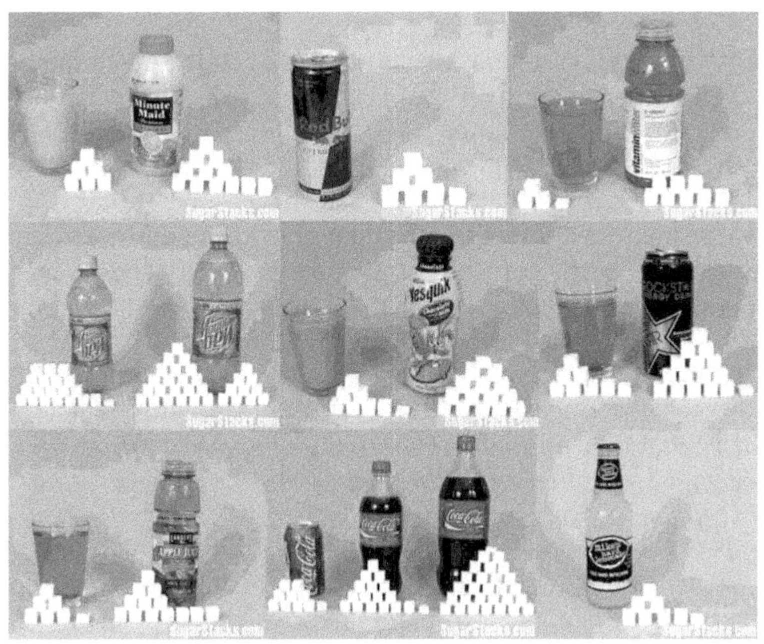

Tip #25
The product that destroys health

Soft drinks truly are the real thing when it comes to playing havoc on not only our nation's obesity epidemic, but also our health crisis.

We as a nation has been brainwashed with the constant barrage of media and TV commercial campaigns promoting all of these sugar in a bottle beverages.

So many people believe that drinking soft drinks are perfectly safe, especially with the constant flood of hip & cool advertisement campaigns constantly entering our brains.

We continue to see happy, lean people drinking these super unhealthy beverages, *but we cannot connect the dots in understanding how terrible this liquid sugar in a can is to our body.*

And by the way, not one of the thousands of soda pop commercials that they have put out over the past 50 years has ever had one fat guy or girl guzzling down one of these poisonous drinks on television or in an advertisement.

All soft drinks are nothing more than poison to your body. A cute little can or bottle of this stuff has anywhere between 9-16 teaspoons of sugar in it.

If that is hard to grasp simply go to your kitchen and pull out your plastic tablespoon and your sugar supply. Now eat 3 - 5 TABLESPOONS of sugar. *This is the amount of sugar that you are getting in one can or bottle of soda pop!*

Now you will have a better understanding of how much sugar that you are consuming in a little innocent can of soda pop. And we wonder why there are so many overweight people (including children) in our nation.

Listen, *the reason why people drink soda pop is for the instant sugar high.* Take out the sugar and these soft drink companies would never sell another can or bottle of this fat producing liquid again.

My advice is to completely stop buying any beverage in a can or bottle unless you want to become fat. 99.9% of any product sold in a can or bottle to drink is seriously bad for your health and belly.

If you must drink something, then stick with either water or sparkling water in order to completely avoid the sugar that is included in all of the other drinks out there.

If you are serious about losing weight, then all of these sugary beverages need to be divorced from your life.

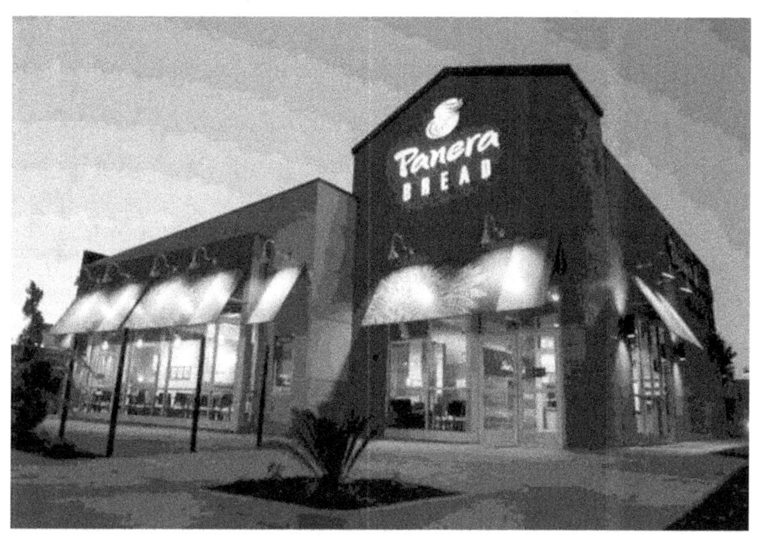

Tip #26
My thoughts on Panera Bread

Who wouldn't like Panera Bread, especially with the warm tan wall colors, fancy lighting, and welcoming fireplace waiting to greet every customer who walks through the door?

I mean let's be real. The yummy goodies and breads at the bakery are pleasant to the eye, and the inside atmosphere is always inviting. Even the bathrooms are clean and up to date.

So seriously, what can possibly be wrong with this popular restaurant with its *cool named sandwiches* and salads? With the great atmosphere and tasty looking food, how can anyone say anything negative about this attractive restaurant?

I personally find the restaurant's overall atmosphere and marketing campaign outstanding. It truly is a warm and inviting place to meet up with friends over lunch. Very few restaurants can compete with their cleanliness, and for that I applaud them.

All of the above gets my thumbs up. But... I personally would avoid approximately 75% of the food items on their menu if I were looking to improve my health or lose weight.

Outside of the salads (which I have no problem with), the rest of the items on the menu are basically made with fat-producing bread.

If you want to seriously improve your health my recommendation is to get all restaurant *(including Panera)* and store bought bread completely out of your life.

You may think you are eating healthy by visiting Panera Bread, but outside of their salads the food being offered is really not healthy for your hips and belly.

It does not matter if bread comes on a fancy white plate or in a pleasant restaurant setting. *Panera Bread will spike your insulin and store unwanted fat around your waistline.*

Do I have anything against this clean and attractive restaurant? Absolutely not, and as mentioned earlier I find the atmosphere to be one of the best when compared to other similar restaurants.

But what I find amusing is how thousands of people honestly think that they are eating healthy whenever they order one of their fancy sandwiches. Remember that *bread is bread is bread* and that includes all of Panera Bread.

Some of you are moaning and groaning right now simply because you absolutely love bread. *But remember, your hips and belly also absolutely loves bread as well.*

Eat the breads and keep the belly, or lose the bread and lose the belly. It is your choice alone.

If you absolutely love Panera Bread and also want to get rid of your belly, my recommendation is to stop eating their breads, fruit drinks, bagels, and ANY bakery item *(sorry gooey cinnamon roll lovers).*

Stick with their salads (without croutons) if you are serious about losing weight.

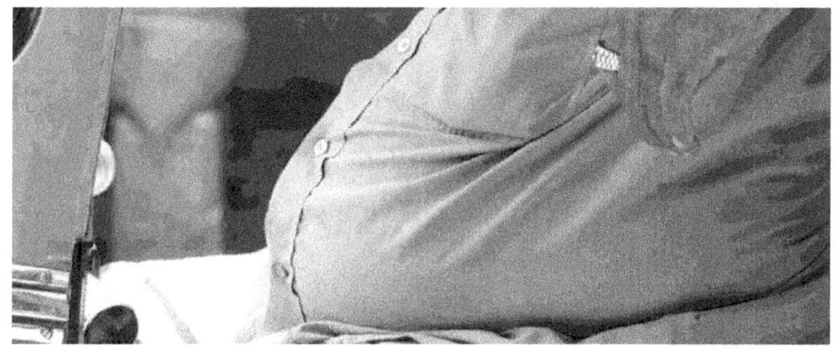

Tip #27
Why are so many people overweight?

Recently I was in a large parking lot waiting for my wife and started to notice people coming in and out of the large department store.

What really caught my attention was the large amount of weight that the majority of people were carrying around their hips and bellies. *It hit me like a ton of brinks how the majority of people in our society are becoming obese.*

And you do not have to be in a parking lot to see this. Go almost anywhere and in any setting where there is a group of people, and at least half of the people you see will be either overweight or obese.

So what is my beef with seeing so much obesity in our society and why should I even care? Great question and here is my answer:

I have a heart for overweight people and what bothers me the most in all of this is that most of these people have no clue on why they are carrying so much extra weight. And more importantly, most obese people have no idea how to lose this extra weight.

Go into any grocery store and you will notice at least 50% of the customers who are shopping are overweight. Now simply look into their shopping carts and you will notice at least half of the products that they are purchasing are unhealthy foods that will continue to make them overweight.

Most of the products in these carts *are cheap processed foods* made in a basement factory. Many are also purchasing a case or two of diet soda pop with the false belief that this will somehow assist them in losing weight.

Being overweight or obese is a by-product of one thing and one thing only...WRONG FOOD CHOICES.

Sure there may be a rare weight disease here and there of why a person is obese, but the majority of people are overweight simply because of their poor food choices that they have made over the years.

Please listen carefully. *You do not have to stay overweight.* You can reverse this if you completely stop putting bad processed food into your belly. Weight will begin to drop by simply learning to eat REAL FOOD.

It is your choice alone, but I am here to tell you that you can lose that weight permanently and regain a healthier and leaner body.

Start eating REAL FOOD and your body will thank you for it.

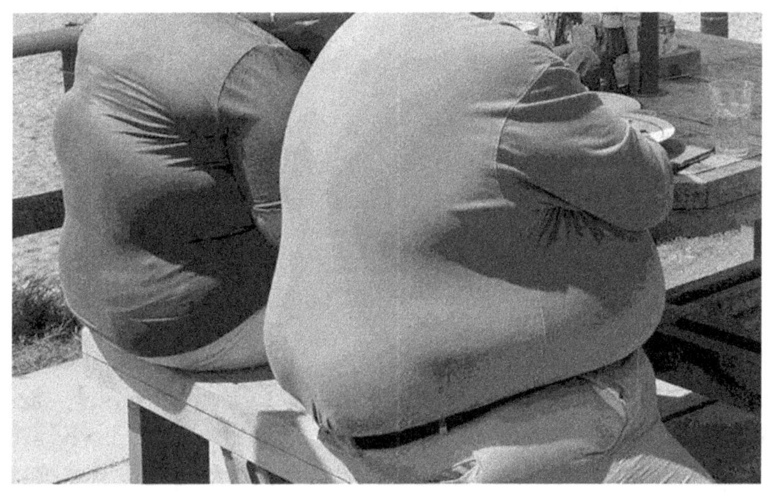

Tip #28
Why do overweight people stay fat?

Outside of the fact that most overweight people are addicted to the fat producing substance we lovingly call sugar, the majority of heavy people simply settle in and "accept" their lot in life.

Let's tackle them both, starting with the toxin known as sugar.

When I speak of sugar, I am not simply talking about that innocent looking white stuff that you buy in a large paper bag at the grocery store.

What I am really talking about is the majority of the products found at your friendly grocery store *since around 80% of these "foods" contain one of the 61 hidden names that sugar goes by.*

Without adding this sweet friend most of these products would sit on a shelf and never be purchased by consumers. *I am also convinced that the #1 product that has contributed to our obesity issue is sugar and all of these processed foods.*

Take away the sugar from your life and weight will begin to drop. Let me say this again in case you may have missed it...

Take away the sugar from your life and weight will begin to drop.

But sad to say, in my personal opinion the majority of overweight people are addicted to this toxin, and have no clue on the amount of sugar that they are consuming each week.

The second major reason that I believe overweight people stay this way is because they have accepted that they are meant to stay fat and cannot see themselves as a leaner person.

I have also come to the conclusion that most overweight people may be afraid of change, especially when it comes to body image. *For some unknown reason we as humans tend to become comfortable where we are, even if it means staying overweight or unhealthy.*

As human beings we tend to be afraid of a major change in our personal life, even if means having a better, healthier life.

I have said this often and will continue to say this...losing weight and keeping weight off takes courage. It is entering an unknown territory of having to adjust to a new, leaner lifestyle.

My advice is to make your life healthier by taking the risk in losing weight and then keeping that weight off. Your new leaner lifestyle will be well worth it.

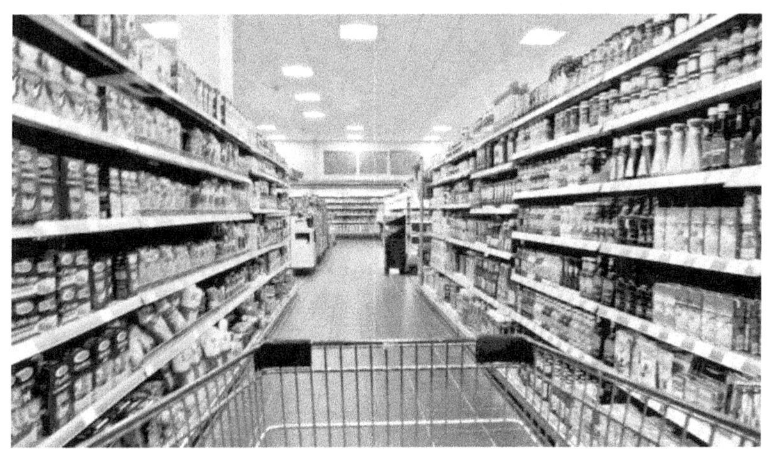

Tip #29
5 foods I stopped buying and what it did for me

Here is a list of five foods that I use to eat regularly. I then began educating myself on how bad each are to my health, and decided to divorce them from my life.

I will also share what quitting these foods did for my health:

#1 CEREALS

It sounds so un-American to ever say anything bad about our beloved boxes of cereals. I mean really, Tony the Tiger and Captain Crunch are about as American as they come.

Grocery stores dedicate a whole aisle to these *dry desserts in a box* breakfast foods, and they are major profits for big business.

Listen, the majority of cereals on the market are nothing more than a sugar dessert in a box and a terrible way to start your day.

For myself, I don't have brain fog anymore simply because I stopped feeding my body and brain this highly concentrated sugar in a box stuff.

#2 ALL PASTAS

If you ever want a quick spare tire around the hips, then all forms of pastas should be your first and foremost go-to food.

Farmers feed cows corn in order to make them fat, but I am pretty sure any pasta would also do the same trick to fatten them up.

Not only have I completely divorced pasta from my life, but I do not miss the sluggish brain fog that pasta always left me with.

#3 FRIED FOODS

Trust me when I say that restaurant fried foods are really super TERRIBLE for your health. Most are cooked in vegetable, corn, or canola oil, which is an excellent source for future illness.

I personally put french fries up there with donuts in regards to a great product for killing your health. Sure they taste great and are always included with your burger, but fries and sugar-laced ketchup are fat producing and will eventually make you sick inside.

Since quitting fried foods I feel like I have so much more energy. My advice is to get all of these greasy foods completely out of your life.

#4 ALL BOTTLED & CANNED DRINKS

Even though this is not a food, it is a major player for quick weight gain and a big belly. If people simply stopped drinking anything sold in a can or a bottle, *their weight would instantly begin to drop.*

The commonality in all of these canned and bottled drinks is either sugar, which instantly raises the insulin and stores fat on the body, or artificial sweeteners, which is as bad as consuming sugar.

I personally only drink water (and sometimes sparkling water) because I recognize the terrible consequences in consuming these sugary drinks.

Again, I never have a sugar rush or brain fog since divorcing all forms of canned or bottled beverages. I also do not miss those little headaches that came after drinking an innocent can of soda pop.

#5 KETCHUP AND BBQ SAUCE

Let me get straight to the point on these 2 popular sauces...they are nothing more than glorified sugar.

One tablespoon of ketchup includes ONE TEASPOON of sugar which is absolutely ridiculous. Both types of sauces are great for those who want to get a fat tummy.

Don't be deceived as these two sauces are tasty simply because of the hidden sugar included.

I use to love BBQ Ribs with the thick sugary sauce dripping from each rib. But those days are gone. My recommendation if you want to improve your health is to avoid both of these sugary sauces at all cost.

Since quitting ketchup and BBQ Sauce I feel so much healthier simply because I am not loading my body with all of this sugar.

"The majority of cereals are nothing more than a sugar dessert in a box and a terrible way to start your day."

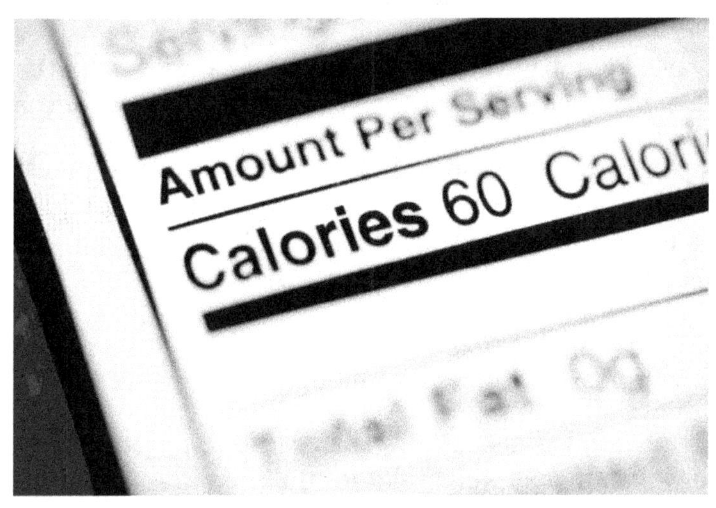

Tip #30
Dieters fail because they count calories

Calorie counting is a total waste of time, and this whole calorie counting thing *is not the answer to healthy weight loss in my opinion.* The vast majority of people on a calorie counting diet eventually fail.

I would tell anyone who wants to lose weight to stop counting calories and learn to eat REAL FOOD *(hello steak & eggs).* All of these diet brand "low calorie" foods on the market are absolutely terrible for your health.

I mean let's be serious. These frozen diet foods brought to you by Jenny Craig, Smart Ones, Nutrisystem, and on and on are nothing more than glorified processed food, and will eventually ruin your health.

And I really don't care if they are "low in calories". If you want to lose weight then you need to stop looking at calories, and simply begin to eat quality food until you are completely satisfied. This is the only safe and permanent way to get fat off of your body.

Listen carefully... you are wasting your time counting calories. The fat on your body has very little to do with calories *and everything to do with the quality of poor food choices that you are making.*

I shake my head in disbelief that people would actually eat a terrible processed fake food like Nutrisystem Lasagna or a chocolate brownie sundae and think that they are eating healthy in the hope of losing weight.

All of these diet programs give people nothing more than unhealthy processed foods, even though it is "low in calories."

I am dumbfounded and utterly amazed that so many people who sincerely want to lose weight fall for this.

What matters the most is THE QUALITY of the food if you want to get back that teeny bopper weight that had left you years ago.

Listen carefully... Give me a 16 oz. steak at 1,227 calories over a 500 calorie dish of Nutrisystem pasta any day of the week.

We have an overweight nation because people are not eating quality food, but following this deceptive calorie belief while they continue to eat unhealthy processed food simply because it is marketed as a "low calorie diet food."

A total joke in my opinion. Again, I'll take five bacon stripes (211 calories) over a sugar laced "100 calorie" yogurt cup any day of the week.

Again, if someone wants to lose some serious weight, I would tell them to stop counting calories, and learn to eat REAL QUALITY FOOD until they are completely satisfied.

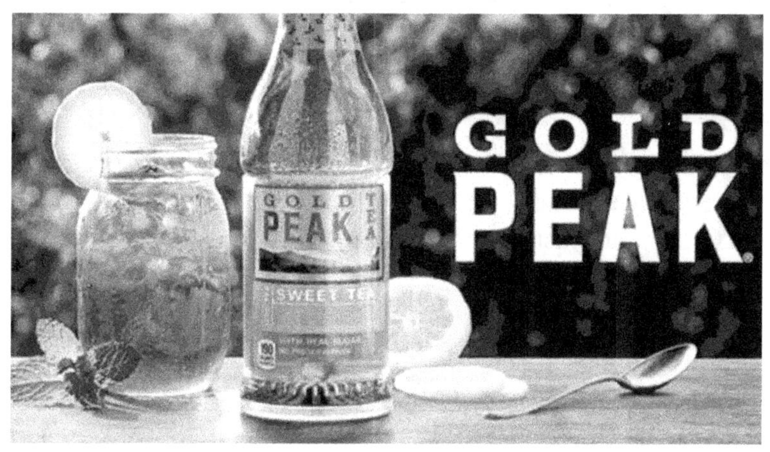

Tip #31
Drink bottled tea products if you want to gain weight

Did you know that the majority of the bottled and canned teas on the market are a great source for putting on unhealthy weight?

Hard to believe but trust me when I say that all of these marketed teas are nothing more than basically sugar water with a little tea included.

It doesn't matter to me if your southern ancestors have been drinking sweet tea for centuries, or if the advertising on the bottle gives the appearance of being a healthy alternative to soda pop. *All of these bottled sweetened teas are terrible for your health and waistline.*

Here is one example... did you know that one innocent 18.5 ounce bottle of Gold Peak has 48 GRAMS OF SUGAR in it. That amounts to 12 teaspoons of sugar in this cute little brown bottle.

You might as well just drink sugar and water and save a couple of bucks from having to buy this unhealthy beverage.

Do not be deceived into believing that any of these teas are healthy. They are all fat producing. *Why would you want to put so much unhealthy sugar into your body?*

And please do not think you are being healthy by drinking one of those diet tea products on the market. The artificial sweeteners they are using are just as damaging to your body as sugar is.

Bottom line... if you are going to drink tea, then keep it at 100% natural with zero added anything except a slice of lemon if you prefer.

Not only will you begin to make yourself healthier, but your body weight will slowly begin to disappear as well.

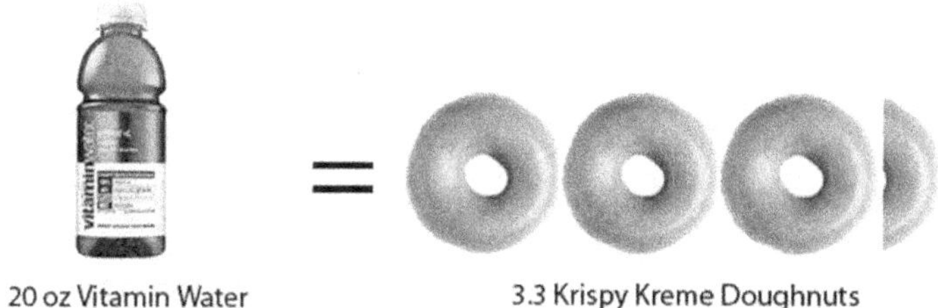

20 oz Vitamin Water   3.3 Krispy Kreme Doughnuts

Tip #32
Vitamin Water is terrible for you

The food and beverage deceptive marketing campaigns continue to give its customers the illusion that most of their processed foods and bottled beverages are good for you.

Here is one example: People buy a bottle of *Vitamin Water* with the naive belief that it must be healthy since the word "Vitamin" is proudly displayed on the bottle.

There is as much sugar in this *terrible for your health* bottled sugar water as 3.3 Krispy Kreme Donuts! Vitamin Water has over 8 teaspoons of sugar included in its bottle.

My advice is to stay away from 99.9% of any beverage that is in a can or bottle unless you want to become unhealthy. Or better yet, simply forgo the Vitamin Water and munch down 3.3 donuts instead.

"The food and beverage deceptive marketing campaigns continue to give its customers the illusion that most processed foods and bottled beverages are good for you."

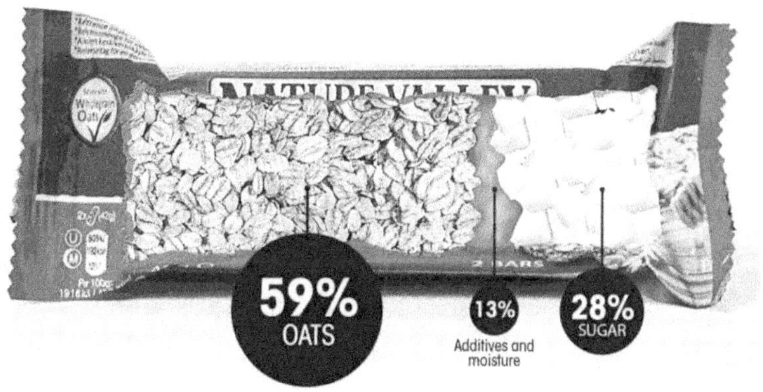

Tip #33
"Health" bars will make you fat

Here is another example of big food corporations fooling the masses with the dozens of so-called health bars that flood your friendly grocery store aisles.

One example of a "health" bar is called *Luna* that I am sure you can easily find at a grocery store. It promotes itself as a healthy alternative when in reality it is nothing more than *an insulin spiking glorified candy bar.*

One Luna Bar has as much sugar as 1.1 Krispy Kreme Donuts, which is absolutely ridiculous.

What bothers me the most about all of this deceptive marketing is that the majority of people who really do want to start becoming healthier or lose weight are deceived into believing that these "health" bars are good for them.

My advice is to not waste your money on what I would consider unhealthy food.

"What bothers me the most about all of this deceptive marketing is that the majority of people who really do want to start becoming healthier or lose weight are deceived into believing that these "health" bars are good for them."

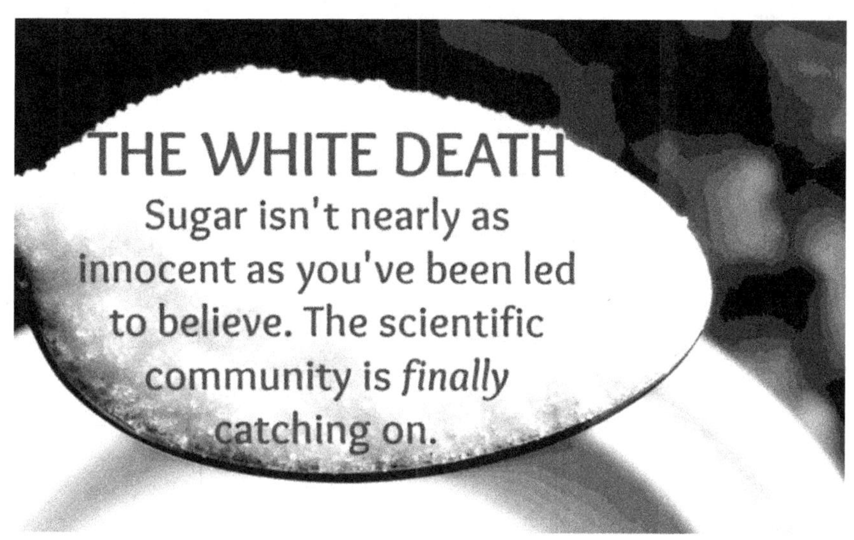

Tip #34
Lose pounds by doing one simple thing

If you have tried every diet under the sun and continue to fail in losing that extra weight, I have a solution *that will work* to permanently become leaner within one short month:

Stop eating all forms of sugar and processed foods (which turn into sugar), and replace it with eating healthy fats.

For just one month begin to eat healthy fats *(just Google it)* instead of sugar and your weight will begin to dissolve. Eating a large percentage of fats in your daily diet will not only keep your insulin low (which is a key to losing body fat), but will also keep you completely full and satisfied for a very long time.

If you are addicted to sugar or refuse to give up your Twinkies, then I really cannot help you. In my opinion, sugar is addicting to most people, is one of the main reasons for our obesity epidemic, and is a major player in our nation's health crisis.

But if you have reached the breaking point of being sick and tired of being overweight, then my advice would be to quit this toxin we affectionately refer to as sugar, and replace it with eating healthy fats every day.

Do this for one month and your friends will begin to take notice. Do this for one year and your friends will not recognize you. Do this for the rest of your life and you will stay at your desired weight.

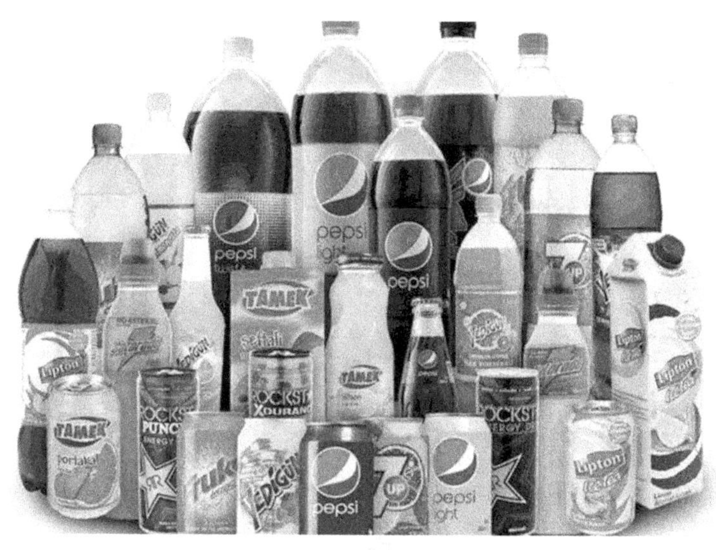

Tip #35
Avoid 99.9% of beverages in a can or a bottle

The vast majority of canned and bottled beverages on the market are nothing more than sugar water with a little favoring.

Drinking these highly addictive sugary beverages is also a major reason that we have become a nation with fat waistlines.

Go to any grocery store and the shelves are lined with dozens of various canned and bottled beverages that are really unhealthy for you.

They also are addicting due to the large amount of added sugar, and have become our favorite source for a quick sugar fix.

Here are a few beverage examples that you need to avoid if you want to become a leaner person. And as mentioned, they are nothing more than sugar water:

#1 ALL SODA POPS (along with all diet pops)

#2 Lemonade Drinks (basically just sugar and flavoring)

#3 Sweet tea (and green tea which is really just sugar water)

#4 ALL FRUIT JUICES (even 100% juices - which convert to sugar)

#5 HOT CHOCOLATE (it is just basically sugar and cocoa)

#6 Apple Cider (hot or cold, and again converts to sugar)

#7 Vitamin Water (it is just a sugar drink as well)

#9 Sport Drinks (Gatorade is a train wreck for your health)

#10 And the myriads of other bottled and canned beverages.

Listen, the reason that all of these beverage products sell is because of *the instant sugar rush* that quickly satisfies the majority of people who are addicted to sugar and do not even know it.

Drink a can of soda pop and you are instantly rewarded with 9 - 16 teaspoons of sugar. *Please understand that it is the large amount of sugar in all of these products that make you crave them.*

You may love that Mountain Dew, but your waistline won't. All of these products will expand your belly, and as an added bonus these sugar-laced beverages will play havoc on your overall health.

My advice if you want to lose some serious weight is to simply withdraw yourself from 99.9% of any beverage in a can or bottle and learn to simply enjoy water again.

Not only will you begin to feel better and think clearer by quitting these sugary drinks, but your waistline will begin to slowly disappear.

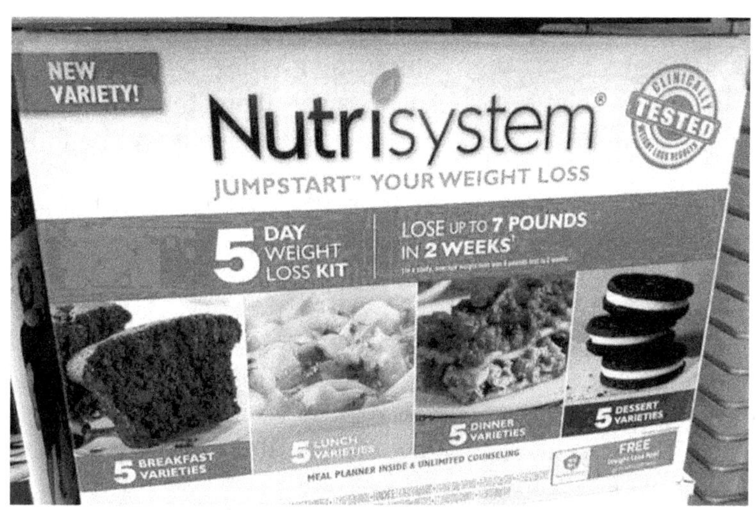

Tip #36
Diet Programs: A complete scam in my opinion

Watch television for any short period of time and you are sure to come across a diet commercial with skinny models trying to scam you into buying a "low calorie" processed food program.

Not only do they entice you to purchase their monthly diet system with those before and after photos of fat people becoming skinny, but they also tempt you with all of the yummy diet foods that will conveniently be shipped to your home.

Let's look at one of the more popular television weight loss programs that spend millions on TV ads to get you on board with them. It's called Nutrisystem.

Every time I see a Nutrisystem commercial with Marie Osmond I laugh inside *and instantly think of the word SCAM.*

Listen, the foods that they will send you if you fork over the cash are really unhealthy for you. I am completely dumbfounded that so many people fall for this.

Don't be scammed by the "calorie myth" since Nutrisystem banks on the brainwashed belief that it is all about the *calories in vs. calories out concept* with no concern for the quality of the food.

In my opinion, losing weight permanently has everything to do with eating QUALITY REAL FOOD that will consistently keep your insulin low throughout the day.

But the foods that Nutrisystem offers are a train wreck in my opinion. I mean let's be real. *How can they promote health by mailing out terrible insulin spiking foods like breads, potatoes, cookies, pizza, brownies, and pastas?* These processed foods are all bad for you.

According to their website, the monthly food plan starts at around $300.00 per month. *You could not pay me that much each month to eat any of this delivered "low-calorie" processed food.*

I believe that all of these diet foods are terrible for your health. And this has nothing to do with Nutrisystem, as I would say this about all of these diet "low calorie" food products being sold.

This also goes for the grocery store frozen "diet foods" that are deceiving people into thinking that they are healthy for you.

Listen, my advice is to stop wasting your hard earned money on all of these processed foods, as the majority of these items will keep your insulin high and eventually ruin your health.

Sure you may lose a few pounds eating this low calorie food, but it will eventually make you unhealthy. And seriously, do you really want to keep forking over money each month for food that I personally would never recommend to anyone?

Bottom line: Run as fast as you can from all of these television diet program scams and simply learn to eat REAL FOOD *(hello steak, eggs, broccoli, and avocados).* Not only will you become healthier, but you will also begin to see weight disappear in a much healthier manner.

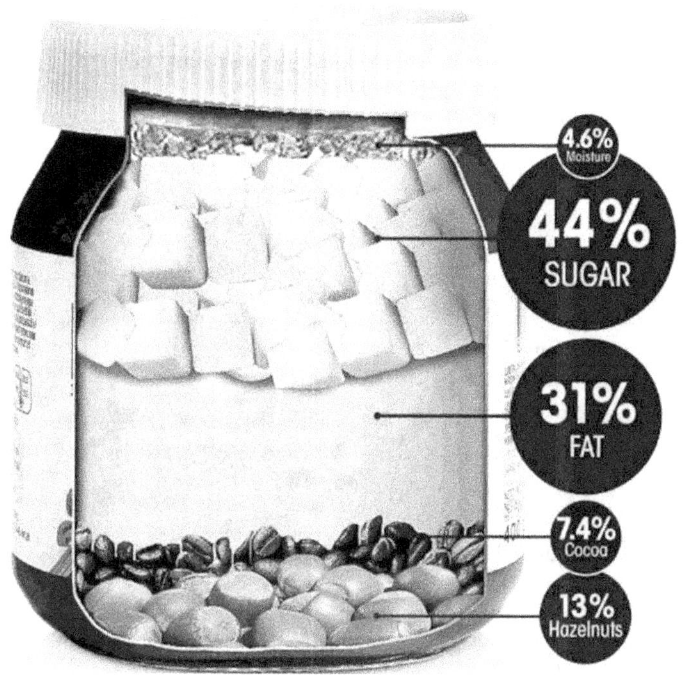

Tip #37
Nutella: You might as well eat chocolate cake frosting

Of all of the products at your friendly grocery store I cannot think of one that is a bigger scam than the product known as Nutella.

It is promoted as a hazelnut spread and gives naive customers the impression that it is a healthy food. *Nothing could be further from the truth.*

This is a total garbage food that will eventually wreak your health and make you fatter. *44% of the jar is nothing but sugar!* No wonder the kids love it.

My advice is to stay far away from this product as well as the other spreads that flood the market, such as jams and jellies that also are laced with sugar. It is important to look at the sugar content in all of these spreads.

Remember that 4 grams of sugar *equals 1 teaspoon of sugar.* So if a product has 32 grams of sugar per serving listed in the ingredients, *it would equate to 8 teaspoons of sugar.*

In my opinion this is a deceptive way to list the sugar content. All ingredient labels *should use teaspoons when listing the sugar content instead of using grams.*

By listing the added sugar as teaspoon measurements, consumers can then easily visualize all of the sugar that they are about to poison their body with.

Read the label and look for the sugar content before buying. Your shrinking hips and belly will thank you for it.

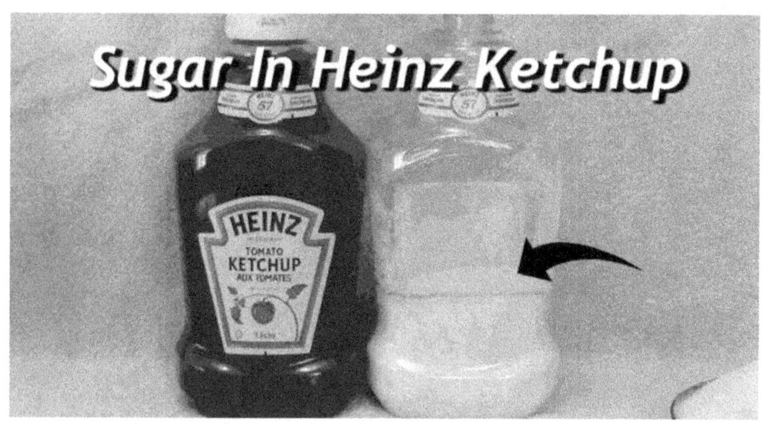

Tip #38
Ketchup is LOADED with sugar

Who in their right mind would ever speak against America's most popular condiment affectionately known as ketchup?

Everyone and their grandmother adore this red gooey stuff. How can Americans live without this condiment, especially for those who douse it on their fat producing french fries?

Let me get straight to the point on the popular product that the majority of Americans have in their refrigerator. *Ketchup is LOADED with sugar.*

Pound for pound it has more sugar than ice cream. If you are serious about becoming leaner, then you need to divorce this red stuff immediately.

For every one tablespoon of ketchup there is ONE TEASPOON OF SUGAR in it! The ingredients include high fructose corn syrup which is seriously damaging to your health and waistline.

My advice is to quit using ketchup along with the sugary BBQ sauces out there if you are serious about becoming a leaner person.

"For every one tablespoon of ketchup there is ONE TEASPOON OF SUGAR in it! The ingredients include high fructose corn syrup which is seriously damaging to your health and waistline."

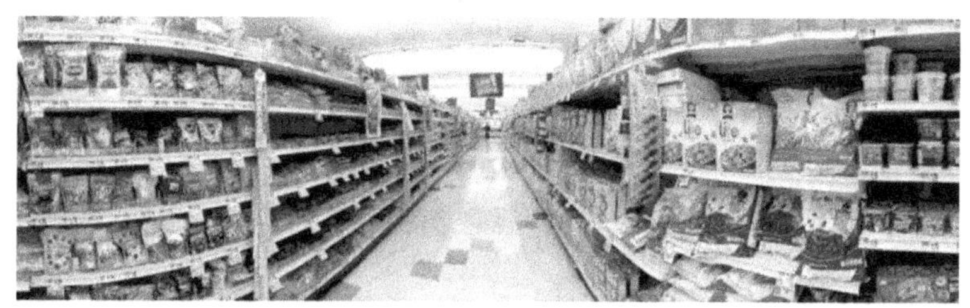

Tip #39
It is a poor diet that has made America fat

I sometimes scratch my head and wonder if there is anyone out there who understands *the simple fact that we have become a fat nation due to our terrible daily food choices.*

Go into any group setting in America and you are sure to find at least 50% of the people within the room either overweight or obese. *There truly is an unhealthy fat epidemic occurring before our very eyes.*

Let me get straight to the point...

Our nation's overweight problem has EVERYTHING TO DO with the 80% of processed foods that are being sold at your friendly local grocery store.

We have been deceived into blindly believing that as long as a grocery store item has a label slapped on it that says FOOD, then it must be safe and healthy to consume.

Listen, the majority of the food items purchased by consumers in any grocery store was either concocted in a laboratory by "food scientists" wearing white coats, or made in a basement factory somewhere in the Bronx.

In other words, it is all processed food and more than likely the major reason that you may be sick or overweight.

Sure it may all taste yummy *(thanks to the added sugar),* but all of this stuff will make your belly and hips expand, as well as put you on medication.

Please understand that our bodies were never meant to consume all of this cheap processed food. Your body eventually rebels by making you fat, and then gives your caring overweight doctor a reason to make extra cash *by putting you on some hard to pronounce expensive prescription drug.*

Listen, stop eating garbage food and you won't need to keep popping those prescription drugs that your doctor keeps giving you. *We as humans were never meant to live off of drugs, period.*

As a side note, the selection of unhealthy foods that most people eat daily simply shows disrespect for the body that they were given. Please also stop fooling yourself into believing *that food is food is food* as long as it is classified *as a food* and sold in a grocery store.

The majority of anything boxed, bagged, canned, or frozen is unhealthy for your body, and again is the main reason that our country has become sick and overweight.

So what is my advice? Stop eating the Standard American Diet (or SAD Diet) *and have the courage to stop shoveling down all of that processed food like everyone else is doing around you.* Be like the crowd and trust me when I say that you will continue to get fat.

Yes, I understand that you have been eating this SAD Diet since you were a little tot. I also was in the same camp and use to adore all of those sugar laced food products.

But if you sincerely want to become a healthy person and lose unwanted weight, *then you really need to start respecting your body more by stop putting all of that processed food down into your belly.*

In the end, it really does comes down to whether or not a person wants to begin respecting his or her body by making wiser food choices.

Change your eating habits and watch your health begin to blossom. Do this, and I can guarantee that your body will reward you by slowly but surely losing that extra weight that you are tired of lugging around.

"We have been deceived into blindly believing that as long as a grocery store item has a label slapped on it that says FOOD, then it must be safe and healthy to consume."

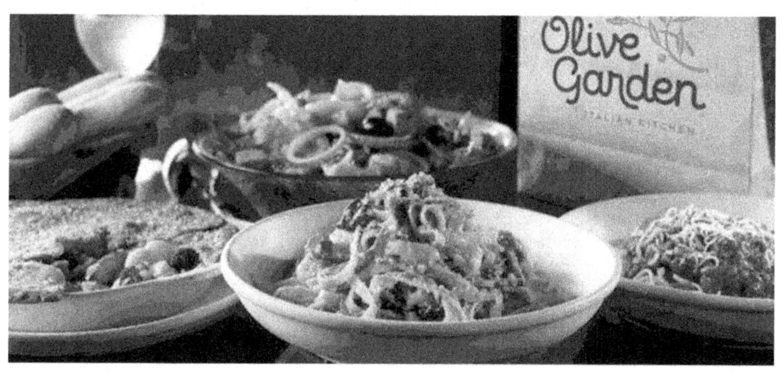

Tip #40
Pasta is a complete train wreck for your hips and belly

We all know that Olive Garden is America's sweetheart when it comes to feeding its fine citizens Italian food.

It is a great place for family and friends to gather, and the ambiance of the restaurant is really quite charming. With nice napkins and fine china, the place is truly welcoming. Even the waiters and waitresses are super pleasant and offer great customer service.

So what is my overall opinion on Olive Garden? I give it super high ratings for its warm atmosphere and great service. It genuinely is a nice place to visit.

But here is why I do not recommend it for those who genuinely want to regain their health and lose those extra pounds...

Pasta is great for putting on extra weight.

Here is the reason why:

When pasta hits your blood stream it instantly converts into sugar, and then raises your insulin *(which is a really bad thing for your health)*. The insulin then stores fat on your body, and as an additional bonus many people get brain fog for a few hours after consuming any type of pasta due to the insulin rush.

I honestly would not recommend any type of pasta and personally view it as an unhealthy food. Sure it has been around for centuries, and yes, there are millions of people who love the stuff.

But this does not erase the fact that from a health viewpoint all forms of pasta *(lasagna, spaghetti, noodles, macaroni, etc.)* instantly convert to sugar and raises your insulin. And for this reason alone I would never recommend pasta for those who are trying to lose weight and regain their health.

All foods that instantly convert to sugar *(breads, potatoes, rice, corn, processed foods)* are terrible for your health. They all instantly raise your insulin, which then does its job of storing fat on your body.

I do understand that there may be times that you will end up at Olive Garden or any of the thousands of other Italian restaurants out there. But remember that consuming pasta should be a rare occurrence in your life if you sincerely want to lose weight.

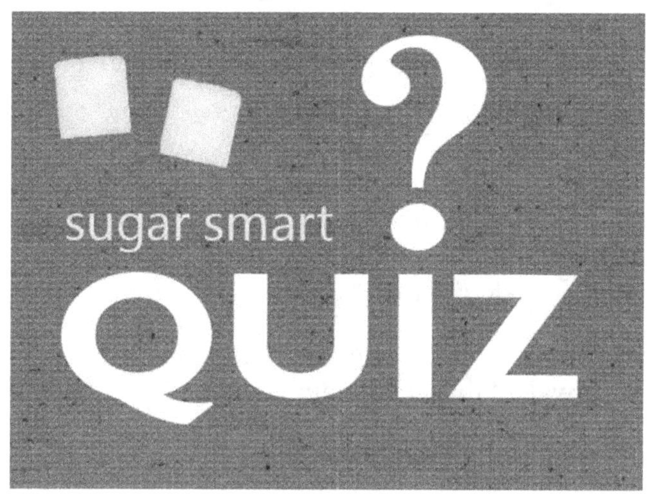

Tip #41
Which food has more sugar?

Here is a quick quiz to test your knowledge on what grocery store item has more sugar…

#1 A Donut or a Can of Tomato Soup?

One can of condensed tomato soup has 24 grams of sugar, while a medium sized doughnut has 18 grams.

#2 Chocolate Candy Bar vs. Dried Cranberries?

A cup of sweetened dried cranberries has a whopping 72 grams of sugar! That's as much as 3-1/2 milk chocolate bars!

#3 Ice Cream vs. Ketchup?

Don't pass the ketchup! Cup vs. cup, ketchup has 21 more grams of sugar than vanilla ice cream.

#4 Canned Pineapple vs. Chocolate Chip Cookie?

Packed in heavy syrup always means that it is loaded with sugar. One cup of canned pineapple in heavy syrup has 43 grams of sugar, compared with 15 grams for a large chocolate chip cookie.

#5 Fruit Smoothie vs. Cupcake?

A 20-ounce commercial fruit smoothie equals 85 grams of sugar. That's more sugar than soda, candy, and a cupcake (37 grams).

#6 Coleslaw vs. Baked Beans?

Both dishes have about 15 grams of added sugar. A one-cup serving is equivalent to a small doughnut.

#7 Gummy Worms vs. Raisins?

A cup of packed raisins has more sugar than any other item in the quiz with 98 grams. Also stay away from the candy as it has over 90 grams per cup!

#8 Soda vs. Grape Juice?

One cup of grape juice has 36 grams of sugar compared with 32 grams in a can of soda *(depending on the soda brand)*.

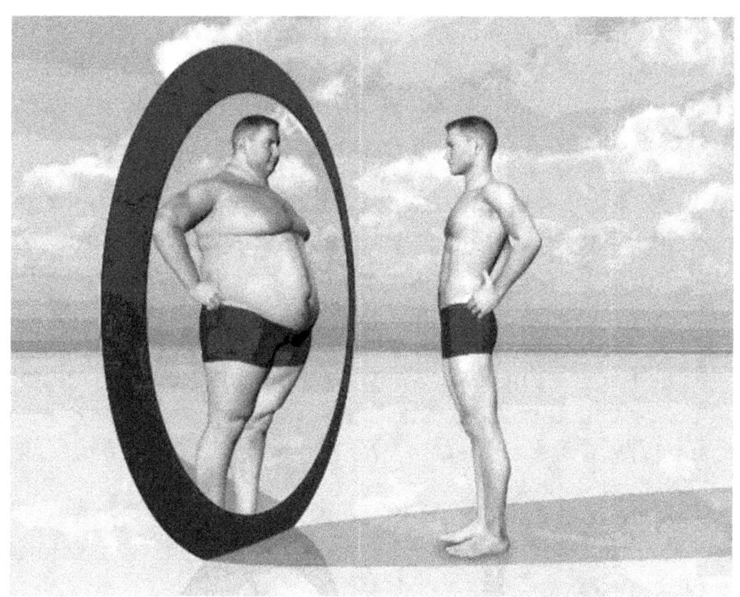

Tip #42
Are you finally fed up with being fat?

1 out of 3 Americans are obese and cannot get to the root cause of why they cannot lose the weight. It not only can become depressing, *but being overweight is not a good place to be health-wise.*

Most overweight people have tried all of the fad diets that come out every month, and still cannot lose the weight that they so desperately want to get rid of.

Other overweight people simply have given up and have accepted that "being a fat person" must be their calling in life.

Let me be straight forward with anyone desperately wanting to lose 10, 20, 50 or 100+ pounds:

Going on a gimmicky diet or a calorie restricting diet will eventually fail you in the long run.

Why? Simply because staying on a calorie deficient diet *eventually becomes unsustainable* (except for those who love to starve themselves).

It may work for 3-4 months with weight coming off, but trust me when I say that you will eventually get sick and tired of this miserable lifestyle *(like the millions before you have)*.

And please stop fooling yourself with all of those silly and goofy diets promising weight loss. They are all scams in my opinion and will not work in the long run. These silly diets all go by goofy names like *The Cookie Diet*, or *The Hollywood Grapefruit Diet*.

I am also amazed that a segment of our society is tricked into wasting their money and purchasing diet pills as the solution to their weight problem.

Again, these are temporary fixes and will not work in permanently keeping the weight off. There is really only one healthy way to lose your belly and hips and here it is:

> *Stop eating sugar and all processed foods that make up approximately 80% of anything in a grocery store.*

Completely make a conscious decision to divorce these fat producing fake foods and learn to simply eat what 'ol Abe Lincoln would have eaten prior to the advent of processed foods... *and that is REAL FOOD.*

Do this and trust me when I say that the weight that you have been carrying around for years *(or decades)* will eventually have to leave.

Totally change your eating lifestyle and watch as your body will eventually begin to lose the weight that you have been carrying around for years. Remember that eating does not make you fat. Eating bad food does.

The enemy to your overweight body is and always has been the poor selection of processed foods that you have stuffed yourself with for so many years.

Have the courage to not follow the crowd and begin treating your body with more respect by giving it REAL FOOD. You will soon be seeing a new person in the mirror staring back at you!

"Remember that eating does not make you fat. Eating bad food does."

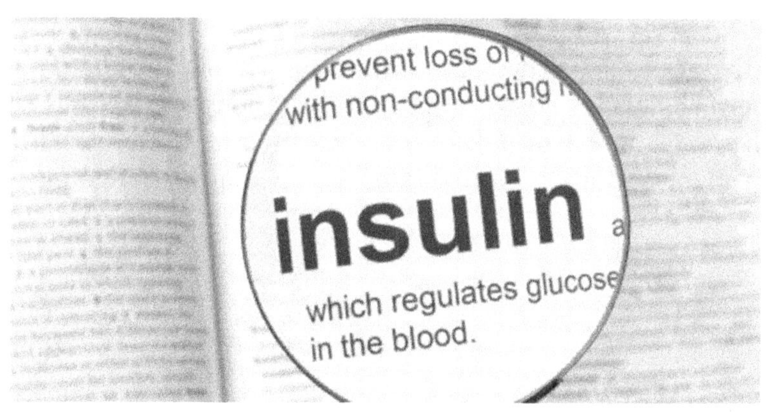

Tip #43
Focus only on ONE THING to lose weight

My advice to anyone reading this who would like to lose weight permanently is to run as fast as you can from the myriads of silly diets out there and just do one thing:

Learn to keep your insulin low throughout the day by eating REAL FOOD.

As mentioned in previous chapters, calorie restriction diets do not work *(think of all of the TV diet commercials out there)* simply because you will eventually get tired of starving yourself and quit after 3-4 months.

So what exactly do I mean *by keeping your insulin low?* Instead of me having to type in what this means and how to keep your insulin low throughout the day, there is an outstanding 26 minute video on YouTube that explains the damaging effects of having high insulin.

If you are looking for that high school weight that you once had but somehow lost over the years *(by following the Standard American Diet, or SAD Diet),* then just spend 26 minutes of your time letting Bob Briggs explain the importance of low insulin.

Simply go to YouTube and watch *Butter Bob - The Root of Modern Illness – High Insulin.* He is a super nice guy from Tennessee whose words I personally would trust more than your overweight doctor who would rather give you prescription pills.

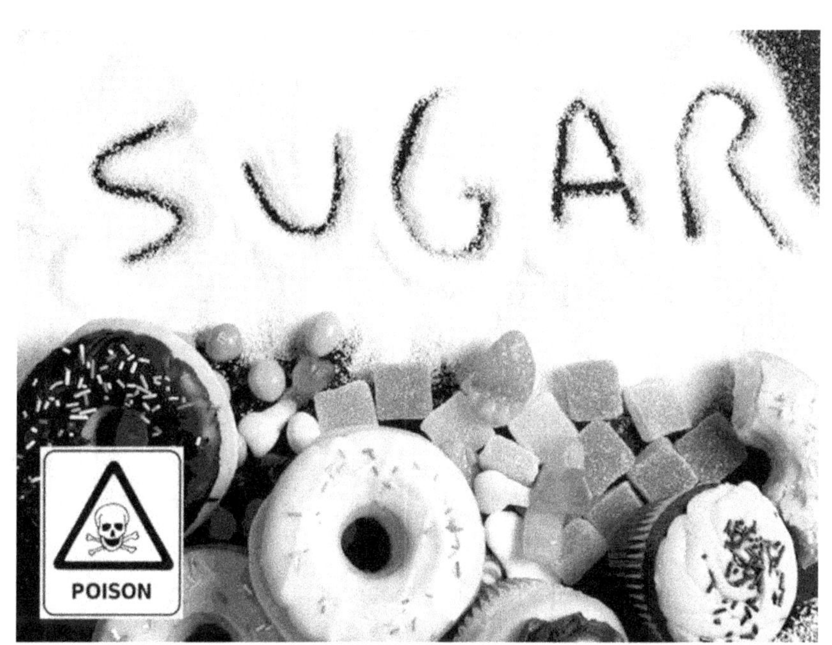

Tip #44
Go 7 days without sugar and watch what happens

Did you know that there is a high percentage of people within our society who are overweight and simply do not believe that sugar has anything to do with it?

Amazing but true.

Either they won't believe it simply because our caring government allows sugar to be put into almost every food product, or they won't believe it *since most people are addicted to this toxin and could never imagine divorcing it.*

Here is the bottom line:

Either keep the constant daily sugar intake and keep the belly, or quit sugar and lose the weight. It's that simple. You cannot lose weight and continue to keep your love affair with this fat producing friend.

So if you are one of the brave few who are fed up with lugging around all of that extra weight, *my simple advice is to flat out quit consuming sugar.* And trust me when I say that more than likely you will feel alone in this journey.

Here is a simple challenge:

For 7 days divorce sugar from your life as well as anything that instantly converts to sugar *(sorry pasta, bread, and all of those processed foods that you may love).* After just one week watch what happens to your brain and belly.

Not only will you begin to think clearer, but your pants will begin to loosen up. *This is all because you stopped eating sugar and processed foods.*

Do this and I can guarantee that you will not only feel better *(goodbye brain fog),* but your body will begin to lose all of that weight that you so desperately want to lose.

Sounds easy doesn't it? But trust me when I again say that it can be a lonely road and difficult to do in our sugar loving society.

But the benefits of living in a healthier and leaner body are so much better than living with brain fog in an overweight body.

Again, you will more than likely be alone in this journey, *but the new leaner person in the mirror will thank you for quitting sugar.*

A final thought... have you ever noticed that people who do go on a "sugar fast diet" for a few days always declares how much better they feel?

My only question is *why do they eventually go back to the toxin that made them unhealthy in the first place?*

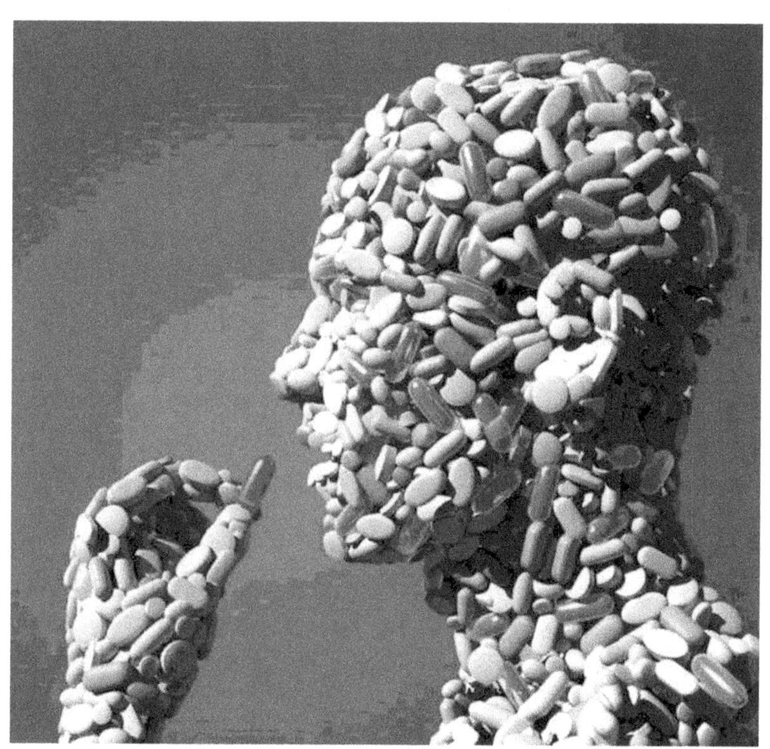

Tip #45
Does a poor diet eventually lead to prescription pills?

I was recently in a Walgreens walking around and noticed an overweight woman in line at the prescription counter waiting for her drugs.

The ironic thing in all of this is that in both of her hands were cartons of ice cream that she was also purchasing.

I would compare this scene to a man heading for surgery for a diseased liver while he is holding two bottles of vodka as he is strolled into the operating room.

I am personally amazed that people cannot connect the dots in the fact that eating garbage food more than likely is a major reason that we have become a nation addicted to prescription drugs.

In my opinion this is nothing short of a travesty as more and more people are relying on prescription drugs.

A large percentage of doctors are giving their patients bandages in the form of a prescription pill without ever asking about their diet.

And like innocent sheep, the majority of people without question trust their doctor's drug recommendation. *I am personally amazed that so many people blindly follow their doctor's advice without questioning anything.*

Most patients will never question why their drug pushing doctor automatically wants to give them a pill to solve the issue without getting to the root of the problem *(which more than likely is a terrible diet).*

Not to bust anyone's bubble, but we were never meant to live off of pills. We've been brainwashed with the hundreds of warm and fuzzy commercials being played every night on television into thinking that it is normal to take prescription drugs.

I really do scratch my head with our ever growing pill swallowing society, and personally don't get it.

Listen, *there are just too many serious side effects with all of these prescription pills that the medical profession loves to pass out.*

My advice is to look at your own diet and maybe see if consistently eating terrible food is the real reason that you are depending on pills to get you through the day.

Hopefully you are not like that overweight lady holding two cartons of ice cream as she waits in line for her prescription drugs. Maybe if she started holding vegetables in her hands she wouldn't have to visit that line anymore.

Again, *we as humans were never meant to depend on*

pharmaceutical drugs in order to function. Try cleaning up your diet by eating REAL FOOD, and just maybe you can say goodbye to being dependent on these dangerous drugs.

"Not to bust anyone's bubble, but we were never meant to live off of pills. We've been brainwashed with the hundreds of warm and fuzzy commercials being played every night on television into thinking that it is normal to take prescription drugs."

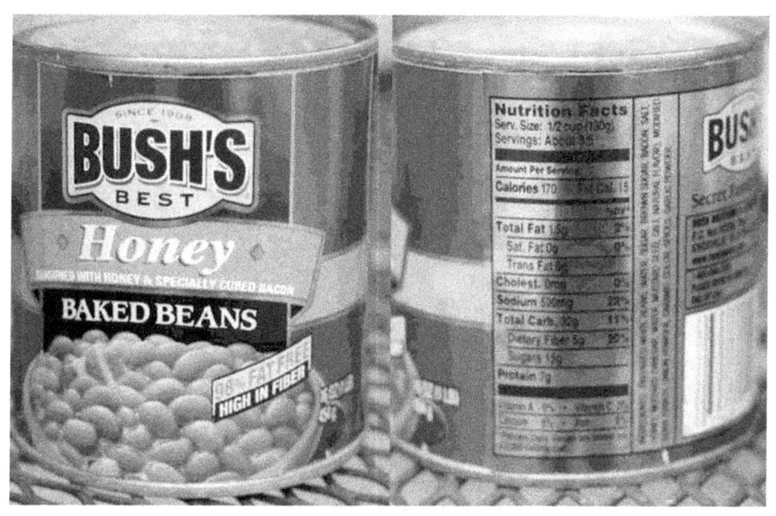

Tip #46
Look for these 2 things on any nutritional list

Let me offer some healthy advice for those who want to begin respecting their body more by feeding it better.

All foods have a nutritional list on the back of the package. Here is my advice on 2 important things to look at:

#1 Look at the SUGAR CONTENT in the food.

The sugar content in any particular food is important since sugar is the main culprit to our nation's obesity epidemic. Remember also that *for every 4 grams listed, it comes out to equal 1 teaspoon of sugar.*

Here is an example: If the Snickers bar you are about to scarf down has a total of 20 grams of sugar, then what it is actually saying is that the bar has a total of 5 teaspoons of sugar in it.

But be careful as some products are very deceptive. If a bottle of sugar ice tea list 25 grams of sugar and the SERVING SIZE happens to be 2, *then you are now consuming 50 grams of sugar.* That bottle of tea has over 12 teaspoons of sugar in it which is great if you want to gain weight.

Keep sugar low and not only will you gain a sharper mind, but your belly and hips will begin to melt away.

#2 Look at Total Carbohydrates

The majority of processed foods are made with cheap refined carbs which are great for expanding the waistline.

My recommendation is to get away from all of those fat producing carbohydrate boxed and bagged grocery store foods. You really should completely cut them out of your life *(sorry junk food lovers)*.

Most Americans eat somewhere between 200-300 grams of carbohydrates each day and we wonder why we have become an obese nation.

I personally try to keep my carb intake to less than 25 grams a day, and honestly have no desire for the hundreds of processed food products at any given grocery store *since I feel in love with REAL FOOD.* Vegetables are my main source for carbs.

Listen carefully. Our bodies were never meant to eat all of these cheap processed carb foods, and it is a major reason that we have become overweight and dependent on prescription drugs.

My recommendation is to divorce all refined carbs and watch what happens to your brain and body. *Trust me when I say that you will feel a whole lot better.*

I personally am not interested in the total calories of a food product as this becomes minor if you are eating REAL FOOD that is not manufactured.

In my opinion this whole calorie thing is a deception because people become fixated on the total calories of an item *and then choose unhealthy "low calorie" processed foods instead.*

If people simply started eating REAL FOOD and stopped worrying so much about calorie counting, we would begin to see a leaner and healthier nation.

Here is one last thought on looking at nutritional labels. I would also recommend to anyone to look at all of the ingredients on the label and see if there is anything that you cannot pronounce.

If you cannot pronounce any of the ingredients listed on the back of the product, then it may be a smart move to avoid purchasing it. Also remember that the more ingredients in a food product, the more processed it is.

With REAL FOOD you will never see a long list of ingredients or words that you cannot pronounce. Look for products that have a short ingredient list, and you will be on your way to a healthier and leaner you!

"*Our bodies WERE NEVER MEANT to eat all of these cheap carb foods and it is a major reason that we have become fat and dependent on prescription drugs.*"

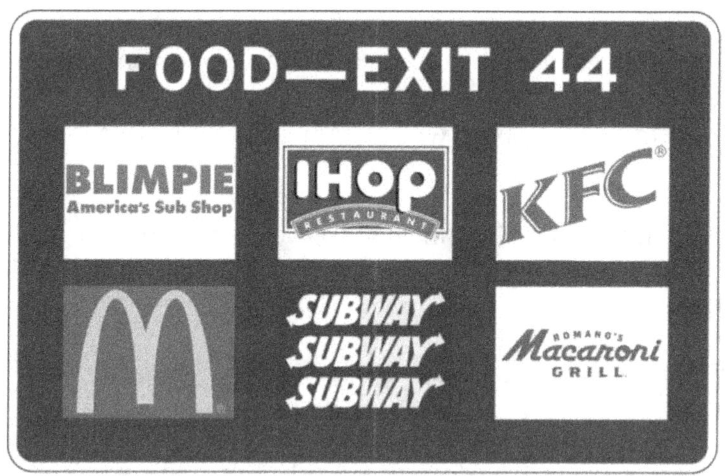

Tip #47
Are you living on a restaurant processed food diet?

If I had to pinpoint another major reason that most of the people in your neighborhood are overweight, I would point directly to restaurants and their boxed processed foods.

With the attraction of being fast and convenient, *a large segment of our population have adopted a lifestyle of depending on restaurant food for their daily sustenance, and then chasing it down with a sugary soda pop.*

Go out into the marketplace or in any group setting and you will soon be surrounded by overweight people who more than likely eat processed restaurant food three to five times a week.

So what is a typical day for overweight people who depend on restaurants to feed them?

For breakfast they may have had a bagel sandwich and orange juice with the erroneous belief that this was a healthy choice *(trust me, it wasn't).*

For lunch they may have gone to a sandwich shop and ordered one of their exotic fat producing bread sandwiches *(with processed meat and cheese),* along with a cup of sodium-laced processed soup.

And then for dinner they may have went to an Italian restaurant and stuffed themselves with insulin spiking pasta and fat producing bread sticks.

Please understand that the above American restaurant staple diet is a great recipe for becoming fat and sick.

Sure it all may have tasted great, but your body will eventually rebel by gaining more and more weight. *This is also why 33% of adults in our nation are obese or morbidly obese (1 out of 3).*

We as a society have been brainwashed into believing that all of these restaurants are somewhat healthy for us. But in reality the majority of the food on a typical restaurant menu is unhealthy.

The secret is to become wise and learn to order food from a menu that is a better choice for your health.

Sometimes it can become difficult, but if you dig deep enough you can find something on the menu that can be halfway decent for your health. I've always said that I can almost always find something on a restaurant menu to eat.

Yes, there have been moments where I have had to bite the bullet with a *not so healthy* menu pick, but the majority of times I have found something that won't shoot up my insulin and give me brain fog for two hours after consuming.

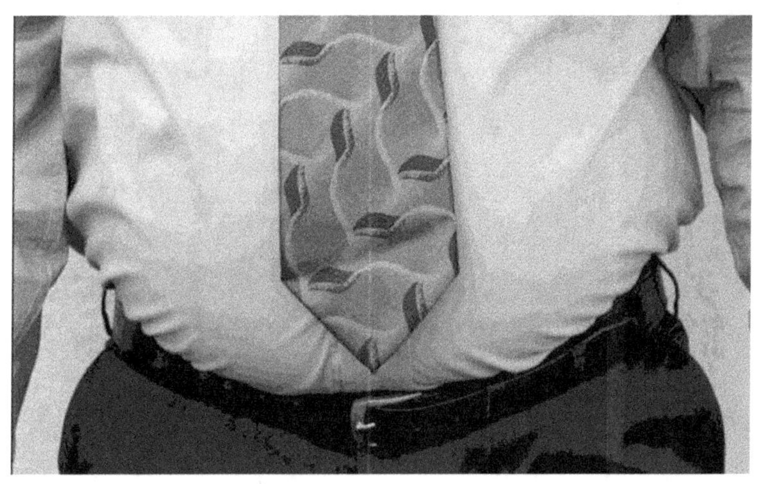

Tip #48
Why do most adult men have big bellies?

Good question and truthfully it has become the norm in our continual feasting society.

In my opinion here is the major reason for this big belly epidemic:

The terrible food selections that have been made for years have finally caught up in the form of a big belly.

In other words, they have lived decades eating anything that is slapped with a label proclaiming that it is a food item *(sorry corn dogs & TV dinners).*

Most men that you see with a big belly were not always like that. In fact some of them actually may have had the exclusive "six pack" in their younger years until gravity and decades of bad food choices finally gave way to a big belly.

For men, the #1 spot on the body that loves to store fat is in the belly region. It is here that the dangerous versical fat makes its home. Big bellies are unhealthy and our belly is usually an accurate reflection of our overall health.

So what is my advice for any guy who wants to lose the belly?

Follow these 3 tips and watch your 46" waist eventually shrink to a 36" waist:

#1 Stop eating sugar and anything that spikes your insulin (think breads, pastas, potatoes, fried foods, chips in a bag, soda pop, etc.).

#2 Make intermittent fasting a daily part of your life (just eat either between 12:00 to 8:00 pm, 12:00 to 6:00 pm, or 2:00 pm to 6:00 pm).

#3 Learn to simply eat REAL FOOD (what 'ol Abe Lincoln may have eaten).

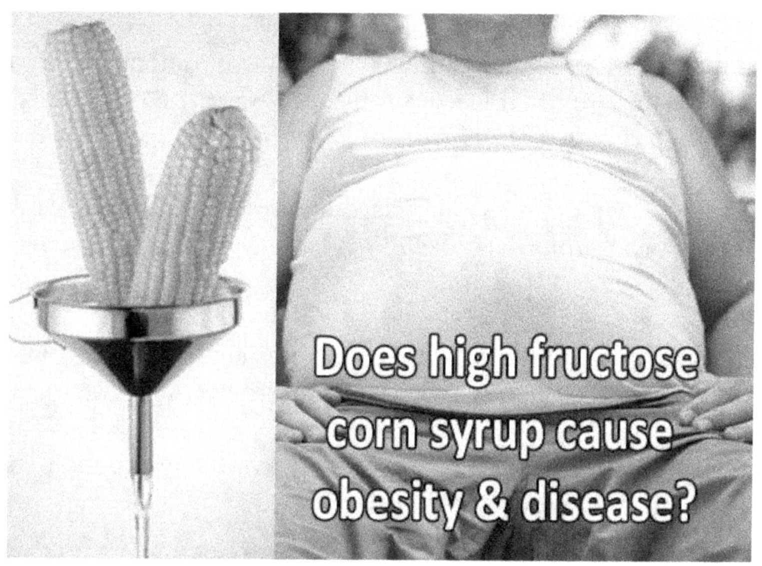

Tip #49
A warning against high fructose corn syrup (HFCS)

Did you know that approximately 80% of the processed foods that we consume contain high fructose corn syrup? According to one definition…

"High fructose corn syrup (HFCS) is a calorie-providing sweetener used to sweeten foods and beverages, particularly processed and store-bought foods. It is made by an enzymatic process from glucose syrup that is derived from corn.

HFCS is a desirable food ingredient for food manufacturers because it is equally as sweet as table sugar, blends well with other foods, helps foods to maintain a longer shelf life, and is less expensive (due to government subsidies on corn) than other sweeteners."

You can now see why companies who produce food and beverages would find the use of HFCS desirable, *but what you cannot see is the potential damage HFCS causes to our bodies.*

The average American has increased their consumption of High Fructose Corn Syrup alone *from zero to over 60 pounds per person per year.*

When used in moderation, HFCS is a major cause of heart disease, obesity, cancer, dementia, liver failure, tooth decay, and more.

Here are 5 reasons why you should try to avoid any products that contain high fructose corn syrup:

1. Ingesting large amounts of sugar, no matter what the form, causes obesity and disease.
2. HFCS and cane sugar aren't processed the same way by the body.
3. HFCS contains contaminants including mercury that aren't regulated or measured by the FDA.
4. Independent medical and nutrition experts don't support the use of HFCS in our diet.
5. HFCS is almost always a marker of food that is lacking in nutrients.

Bottom line:

- *Avoid any products containing high fructose corn syrup or added fructose, which have many negative health effects on the body.*

- *High fructose corn syrup definitely tops the list of health-hazardous ingredients to avoid as much as humanly possible.*

STOP COUNTING CALORIES TO LOSE WEIGHT

Tip #50
Stop counting calories if you want to lose weight

As a follow up to an earlier chapter on calorie counting, here is a reminder if you want to become leaner:

Never think about the word calorie again.

As previously mentioned, this whole calorie scam has made billions of dollars for the diet industry *(Weight Watchers, Jenny Craig, Nutrisystem, etc.)* along with brainwashing everyone into thinking that their weight problem has everything to do with eating to many calories.

So what does everyone do in their attempt to lose weight?

#1 They restrict food (calorie) intake

#2 They feel miserable after a few months

#3 They lower their metabolism

#4 They lose muscle tone

#5 They eat unhealthy "low calorie" food

#6 They eventually quit and gain back the weight

Oh, and by the way, most people on these calorie restricting diets will gain more weight than they had when they originally started their low calorie diet.

The real problem has nothing to do with this concept called calories and everything to do with consuming poor quality food.

I personally believe that being overweight has everything to do with all of the processed, refined junk food that people are putting into their bellies every day.

If you want to permanently become a lean person then my recommendation is to totally get rid of all of the CARBage that you are eating. *Listen, your body does not need these carbs to function.*

The problem with the majority of overweight people is that they are living off an incredible high amount of unhealthy processed carbs each day (200-300 grams a day). This is also one of the reasons that most people feel tired and get brain fog.

Not to burst anyone's bubble, but our body was never meant to eat so many processed carbs, and in my opinion this is a major reason that so many people are overweight and unhealthy.

Remember also that these cheap carbs instantly convert to sugar in your body. My advice is to get off of this "calorie kick" since it really has not worked for the majority of dieters for the past 40 years.

Learn to eat foods that keep your insulin low. I call it REAL FOOD *(hello steak and broccoli)*. If you want carbs then stop getting them from foods like bread, corn, and pasta. Start eating vegetables instead.

As I have often said, calorie counting is a total waste of time.

Remember, *it is the quality of the food that matters the most if you are serious about losing weight.*

And as mentioned in an earlier chapter, I would rather eat a 16 oz. 1,227 calorie marbled-laced steak over a 500 calorie pasta dinner if I wanted to stay lean.

"The problem with the majority of overweight people is that they are living off an incredible high amount of unhealthy processed carbs each day (200-300 grams a day)."

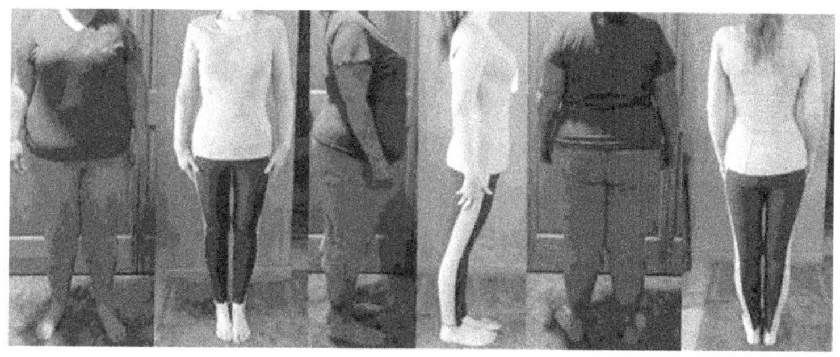

Tip #51
How can I get a flat belly?

Have you ever wondered why the first place that fat likes to settle down into is usually in the belly region? Look at the majority of people over 40 *(or is it 30?),* and most have an overweight belly issue.

So what is the deal, and more importantly, how can you get rid of it in a safe and permanent manner?

Let me give you the reason as well as the solution to obtaining a flat belly.

First of all, underneath our belly region are all of these vital organs. In my opinion, fat loves to accumulate and make its home in this area simply because *it wants to protect all of those vital organs inside our body.*

I also believe that this is the reason that it is usually *the last fat* to want to leave our body.

When a person begins to lose weight, the first areas that will be noticed are usually in the face and arms. *So it is absolutely important to have patience with that stubborn belly fat that will try to stick around for as long as possible.*

So what would be my advice in losing all of that fat and getting a flatter stomach? Here are 3 tips that will do the trick.

#1 Learn to keep your insulin low by eating foods that do not convert instantly to sugar (sorry pastas, breads, & processed foods). By having low insulin you now allow your body to burn body fat as its daily energy source.

#2 Eat REAL FOOD. Choose foods like steak, eggs, & broccoli over pastas, boxed junk, and breads.

#3 Intermittent Fast. Simply eat either between 12:00 pm to 8:00 pm, 12:00 pm to 6:00 pm, or 2:00 pm to 6:00 pm. It means just skipping breakfast (which you do not need by the way).

Intermittent fasting will give your body 16-20 hours of rest so you can then begin to burn that belly fat as your daily energy source.

Just make sure that you eat REAL FOOD and eat until you are full during your eating window. That way you will not be hungry during those 16-20 hours of not eating.

Do the above 3 tips and I guarantee that your belly fat will begin to be burned and used as your daily energy source.

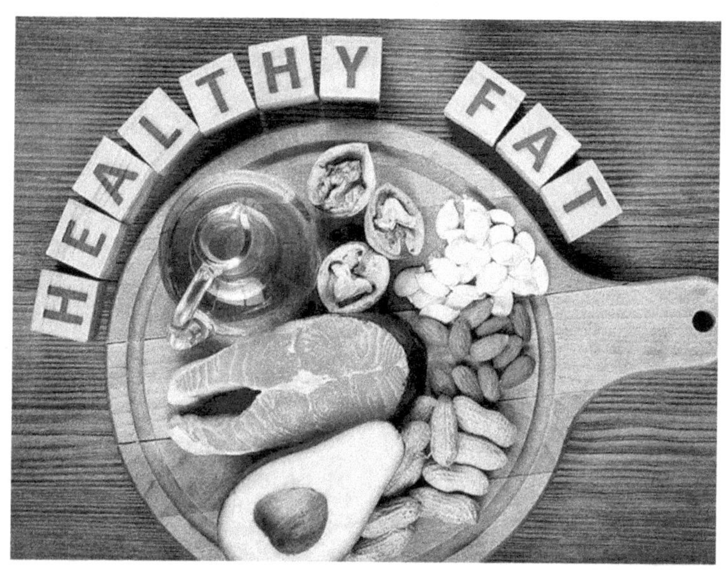

Tip #52
Start eating fat if you want to get lean

Most adults in our nation has been brainwashed for decades into believing that fats are the real enemy and the reason that people become fat.

Let me set the record straight...

The real enemy to getting fat, having heart disease, cholesterol issues, and a host of other chronic diseases is consuming sugar and processed foods.

Let me say that again... Your addiction to sugar and manufactured foods are the real culprit to the majority of health issues. It is sugar that has given us an overweight generation.

What your body is craving and needs is healthy fats. Fats are your friend, unless of course it is trans fats which does major damage to your body *(sorry greasy french fries)*.

Make fats *(think steak, coconut oil, avocados, and hamburger without the bun)* a major part of your food lifestyle and you will lose weight.

I recently came across a book entitled *Eat Meat and Stop Jogging.* It is a great title and so true for those who want to lose weight.

From personal experience eating a diet that is high in fat is the absolute best way to not only lose weight, *but also gain a much more laser-focused brain.*

I like to tell people that I take a multi-vitamin every day, and it's called a steak. Trust me when I say that your brain and body will thank you if you simply get rid of processed foods *(converts to sugar)* from your diet, and replace it with good old fashioned healthy fats.

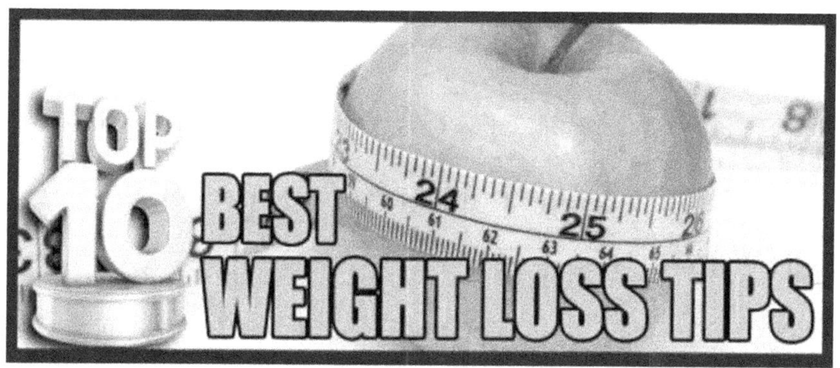

Tip #53
10 of my favorite tips for losing weight permanently

In review, if I had to narrow it down to my favorite top 10 tips for permanent weight loss, the following would be my choices:

#1 FAVORITE TIP:

Understand that *keeping your Insulin low* is the key for allowing your body to burn fat as your main energy source. The only way to do this is by eating healthy foods and avoiding sugar and processed foods.

#2 FAVORITE TIP:

Start eating REAL FOOD and avoid all processed foods *(which make up around 80% of grocery store items.)* If Abe Lincoln could not recognize it, then more than likely it is not real food.

#3 FAVORITE TIP:

Make intermittent fasting a daily part of your life by eating between a 4-8 hour window every day. Simply skip breakfast and you will achieve this. *The 16-20 hour rest from food now prolongs your body to burn its own fat as energy.*

#4 FAVORITE TIP:

Sugar and anything that instantly converts to sugar in the body *(think processed foods)* is the reason most people are overweight. Quit sugar and your weight will instantly begin to drop.

#5 FAVORITE TIP:

Body fat is stored energy waiting to be used. Remember that keeping your insulin low by eating REAL FOOD *(and avoiding bad carbs),* along with intermittent fasting allows you to burn fat as energy. This is the key to losing weight.

#6 FAVORITE TIP:

Try to make your daily diet consist in the area of 70% healthy fats, 25% protein, and 5% healthy carbs. Remember that one of the major reasons why we have an obese nation *is because most people live off of 60-70% of processed carbs every day.*

#7 FAVORITE TIP:

Avoid the majority of products at your friendly grocery store that are boxed, bagged, canned, or frozen. Remember that most of these yummy "made in a factory" processed foods not only keeps your insulin high, but eventually will make you overweight.

#8 FAVORITE TIP:

Avoid 99.9% of any beverage sold in a can or bottle as the vast majority are loaded with sugar or a fake sweetener. *Most of these products are nothing more than sugar water with a little flavoring.*

#9 FAVORITE TIP:

Stop calorie counting and learn to simply eat REAL *FOOD (hello steak & broccoli)* if you want to lose weight. Remember that it is the QUALITY OF THE FOOD that matters the most. Eating does not make you fat. Eating bad food does.

#10 FAVORITE TIP:

It is you and you alone who will make the final decision on your food choices. Choose REAL FOODS that keep your insulin low throughout the day and you will lose weight. Choose processed foods that keep your insulin high throughout the day and you will gain weight.

#11 BONUS TIP:

Weight loss occurs in the kitchen, not the gym. Exercising your body has many positive benefits, but losing weight is not one of them. Sure you may lose a few pounds, *but 90% of serious weight loss occurs only in the kitchen.*

"Body fat is stored energy waiting to be used. Remember that keeping your insulin low by eating REAL FOOD (and avoiding bad carbs), along with intermittent fasting allows you to burn fat as energy. This is the key to losing weight."

Additional Resources

Here are a few additional online resources:

www.dietdoctor.com

This is an outstanding website with 100's of great resources on the low carb lifestyle.

Butter Bob Briggs

www.buttermakesyourpantsfalloff.com

Butter Bob was the person who opened my eyes to the importance of putting fats back into our diets and the importance of keeping our insulin low.

Bob has some outstanding videos online. My recommendation would to go to www.youtube.com and watch these five videos to learn more:

Butter Bob Must Watch YouTube Video Titles:

Butter Makes Your Pants Fall Off (29:02)

The Root of Modern Illness – High Insulin (25:56)

At the Store with Butter Bob (14:22)

You Got to Get Sugar Out of Your Life (13:56)

You are Either Fed or Fasted (9:29)

Check out a few other great YouTube video presenters:

Dr. Robert H. Lustig

Sugar: The Bitter Truth (129:00)

Dr. Eric Berg

The Road to a Leaner You

Dr. Eric Westman

Dr. Jason Fung

Dr. Andreas Eenfeldt

Dr. Tim Noakes

Gary Taubes

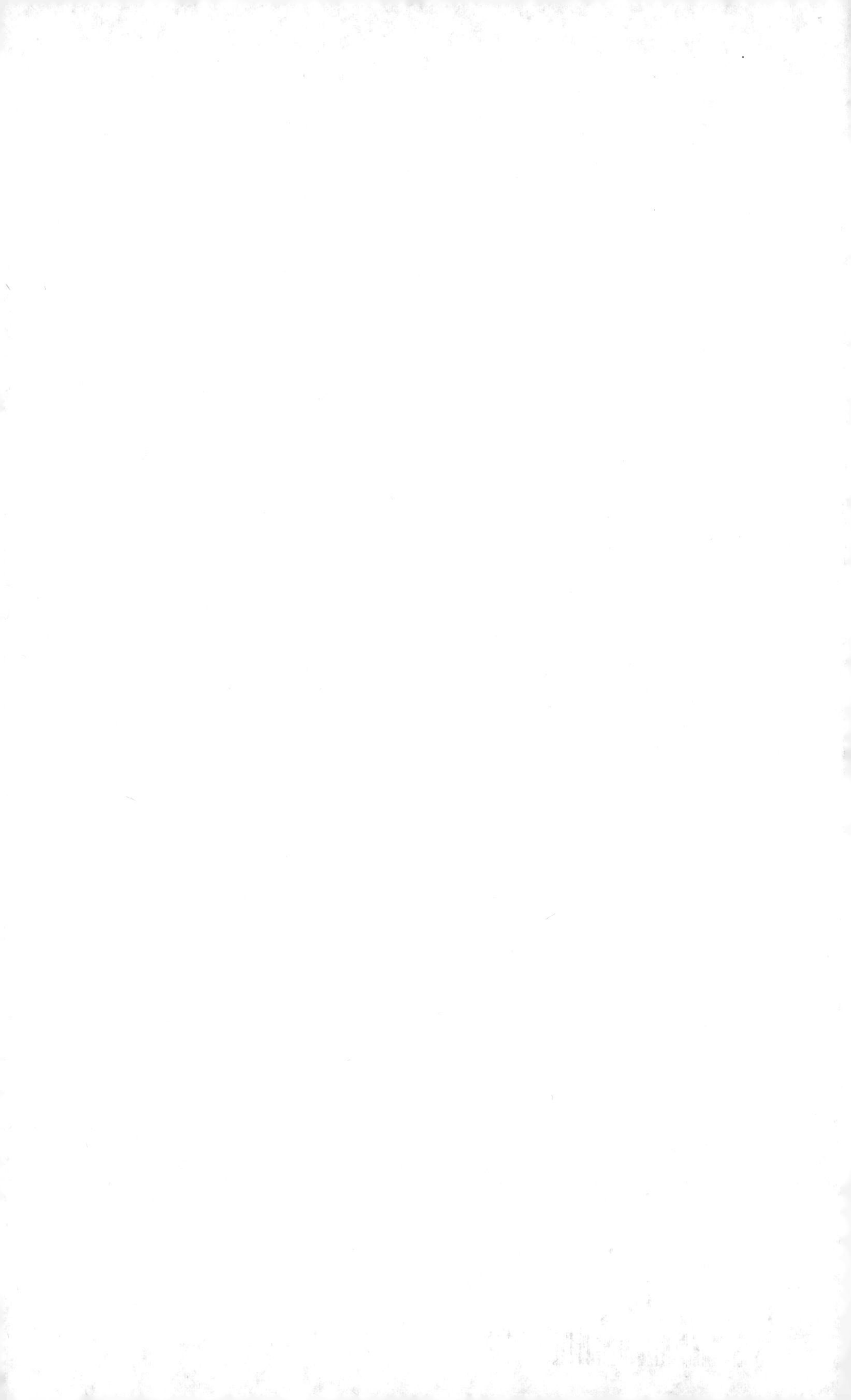